THE CHILD'S UNCONSCIOUS
MIND

Founded by C. K. Ogden

The International Library of Psychology

DEVELOPMENTAL PSYCHOLOGY
In 32 Volumes

THE CHILD'S UNCONSCIOUS MIND

The Relations of Psychoanalysis to Education

WILFRID LAY

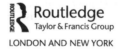
Routledge
Taylor & Francis Group

LONDON AND NEW YORK

First published in 1919 by
Routledge

Reprinted in 1999, 2001 by
Routledge
2 Park Square, Milton Park, Abingdon, Oxfordshire OX14 4RN
711 Third Avenue, New York, NY 10017
Transferred to Digital Printing 2007

Routledge is an imprint of the Taylor & Francis Group, an informa business

First issued in paperback 2013

The publishers have made every effort to contact authors/copyright holders
of the works reprinted in the *International Library of Psychology*.
This has not been possible in every case, however, and we would
welcome correspondence from those individuals/companies
we have been unable to trace.

These reprints are taken from original copies of each book. In many cases
the condition of these originals is not perfect. The publisher has gone to
great lengths to ensure the quality of these reprints, but wishes to point
out that certain characteristics of the original copies will, of necessity, be
apparent in reprints thereof.

British Library Cataloguing in Publication Data
A CIP catalogue record for this book
is available from the British Library

The Child's Unconscious Mind
ISBN13: 978-0-415-20994-6 (hbk)
ISBN13: 978-0-415-86884-6 (pbk)
Developmental Psychology: 32 Volumes
ISBN13: 978-0-415-21128-4
The International Library of Psychology: 204 Volumes
ISBN13: 978-0-415-19132-7

CONTENTS

CONTENTS

THE CHILD'S UNCONSCIOUS MIND

CHAPTER I

INTRODUCTION

A DEEPER knowledge than ever before is now possible concerning the nature of the child, and with it the nature of the problems of education. By virtue of the new knowledge education becomes more nearly a science than it has been in the past. The new knowledge is a knowledge of a hitherto unexplored, or at least unsuccessfully explored, stratum of the mind, as evident in the child as in the adult, and in the child more controllable than in the adult, because more fluent, less fixed and crystallized. We knew that children were, in general, more educable than adults. Now we know the true cause why, and also why some children are more educable than others, and why some children do better in school than others, or learn as easily in school as they do in life.

The method of the newer psychology, which is that of modern science, is the formation and working out of an hypothesis, testing it daily with all the phenomena that do not fit into older hypotheses, and ultimately giving it up, if another theory more inclusive is found. The hypothesis adopted in the newer psychology, which is that

tentatively presented here as a basis for a newer science
of education, is the hypothesis that the *unconscious portion* of each human mind, child or adult, is an activity
which plays an extremely important, if not an exclusively
controlling, rôle in the life of every individual.

The results of a scientific method of testing this hypothesis leave nothing, so far, to be desired.   Language
alone is found defective, at times, to give a universally
comprehensible account of the conclusions which are
reached.   But it is the belief of the present writer that
so much of value for education, so much that is almost
imperative for parents and teachers, and even older children to take into account, has been recently discovered,
that it is quite time for an attempt to be made to put
this new point of view before all those concerned in the
bringing up of children.   And at no previous time in the
history of mankind has there been so great a need for
radical knowledge of mankind as in a time following
almost universal war.

The object-matter of the newer knowledge is infinitely broader than any ever studied by the same methods
before.   I say by the same methods, because the existence
of unconscious mental activity has been guessed for ages,
and human conduct has always been motivated by the
unconscious desires; but no conscious cognizance has been
taken of it except in a very indefinite and unproductive
way.

The object-matter of the newer knowledge is the
human organism and its modes of functioning, *including the unconscious thoughts* upon which before the present time no really scientific observations have been made.
Whether we regard the human organism, with the acts

and thoughts which express its functioning, as purely physical or purely psychical seems to me to make no difference, if we suppose, as we must, that the same natural laws are found to exist in both. There do appear, to be sure, activities which seem predominantly physical, but it would be difficult or impossible to think away the mental element of such activities; and there are activities which are apparently purely mental, but it is impossible to believe that they are really entirely disconnected from what we call physical conditions.

As examples of what might be taken as purely physical, because not apparently caused by any conscious thoughts, there are the instinctive acts, to which we do not attribute any consciousness in animals, because we do not notice any in ourselves. Mention will be made later of the instincts under two heads of self-preservative and race-preservative.

The modes of functioning of the human organism, taken *in toto* as both mental and physical at the same time, and as including both their conscious and unconscious manifestations, may be regarded descriptively and dynamically. But the description of a state and the narration of an act are both needed in the account of any human condition at any time. I shall be very little concerned with the descriptive end of this matter, except in so far as previous psychology may have been inadequate in its account. The current conceptions of the senses, of perception and of the emotions may have to be added to, in order to include the unconscious in the reckoning.

The problem of education in general, whether academic or other, cannot be adequately solved without including consideration of the unconscious, and the means of education in schools will have to be amplified in order to take in this factor which is now almost universally ignored or " wished onto" fate.

The specific problems are those which touch at the present time, and with the present school equipment and management, the relations between the work, the child, the teacher and the parent. In this we deal with concrete realities and interests which are, from whatever angle viewed, admittedly vital.

The Point of View

In order to get the point of view of the most modern analytic psychology, a view from an angle from which education has so far been very little regarded, it will be necessary for the reader to accept the fundamental postulate of the newer psychology and frankly admit the existence in each and every human of an unconscious (sometimes called subconscious and sometimes co-conscious) mentality. This implies not only that each one of us has mental states that never enter consciousness but also that these unconscious mental states are not only states or conditions or dispositions, arrangements of something inert, but are *activities*, energies or groups of forces which are operating by mechanisms of which only the special student knows anything definite at all. The ordinary person knows practically nothing of the detailed working of these activities, but in his own everyday life he has frequent examples of the conscious results produced by these elaborate and complicated mechanisms.

If we do not know the least thing about the part of the

mind below the horizon of consciousness, below the ter-
restrial surface above which alone our consciousness is
able to see what is going on in full view, yet we have many
times wondered, most of us, what is beyond that visible
horizon or what is the nature of the basis on which our
consciousness sports here and there, like an animate being
on the face of the earth, and on which we build our mental
and intellectual structures. The architect of a real building knows what kind of soil the foundations are in, and
makes different arrangements, according to whether he is
building on sand or rock, or whether, as in the case of
a well-known New York City hotel, a subterranean river
has to be provided with an artificial course under the sub-
cellar.

One of the commonest illustrations of the flexibility or
fluidity of the substratum on which our mental life is built
is the ordinary everyday blunder.* When such a blunder
involves loss of money or injury to person or property, one
frequently hears the blunderer repeat to himself: " I can't
imagine how I ever could have done that! What power
got hold of me to make me so careless as not to see that
that very thing was most likely to happen? "

In a number of these blunders, particularly where there
is no great loss of any kind, the operating cause of the
mistake is easily seen, and most people will readily admit
that it is caused by an unconscious desire or tendency to do
the very thing that was done, or leave undone the very
thing that one forgets to do.

A person makes an engagement with another person,

---

* A careful study of almost any blunder shows first that an activity is
responsible for it, an activity with which our familiar consciousness had
nothing whatever to do.

but does not really wish to keep the appointment. He either forgets it, or absent-mindedly puts himself in a position where it is impossible for him to keep it. For instance, with the conscious purpose of taking dinner with a friend in a suburb, I get ready and go down to the station and find either that I have missed the last train which would get me there in time for dinner, or, by some unaccountable (?) mental freak, have left my money and my check book at home. With conscious irritation but with unconscious satisfaction I give it up, and go back to my real interests. That is, if I have not totally forgotten the engagement or misplaced it mentally to the following day, also a common error.

A blunder of my own shows in an unmistakable way the operation of the unconscious wish.

I went to a department store and bought $27.47 worth of goods and asked to have them charged to my deposit account. After reaching home I was informed by my wife that she had used it up and I had but a dollar or so on deposit there. I immediately wrote a check for $30.00 and mailed it, on the supposition that they would send the goods with a note stating that I had overdrawn. Instead they sent the goods collect on delivery. I asked the driver if he could take a check. As he consented, I left him at the door, wrote a check to R. H. Mercer & Company, for $27.47 and handed it to the driver. He looked at it to see if it was correct, put it in his book, receipted the bill and departed. The next day a special messenger came from Mercer's with the check, and asked if I had received the goods and had written that check. I had not signed it! WHY? Unconsciously I had not wished to pay twice or even to do anything that looked like paying twice. I should have been much surprised, and possibly annoyed at myself, had I been unacquainted with the fact that wishes play so important a part in the actions of every one of us. It is needless to say that at the time I was totally unaware that I had not signed the check. I never should have supposed that with a driver from a large New York store I could get away with a trick like that.

This unconscious omission on my part is a very good example of an omission caused by the unconscious part of my personality. This unconscious factor is an element in the constitution of every normal human mind. Its nature is described in one word: desire. It constantly desires my superiority to my fellow-men in all the relations of life. It has been compared to a current of power which is forever flowing and ready to be applied to any purpose for which the human body is a suitable machine. But it lives on the gratification which comes from the worsting of any contestant, and in a certain sense everything with which and everyone with whom I come in contact is taken by it as a possible or actual rival. It feeds on a feeling of power which it gets by making me overcome or outwit my adversaries. If I do not think of this or that man as an opponent, my unconscious factor does, and makes me unconscious for a brief moment. Of course I was unconscious to a small degree when I forgot to sign my name to that check. I was not in a complete trance, nor did I faint. So was the driver unconscious when he looked at the check and forgot to note that it was unsigned. Neither did he faint nor fall in a trance. He simply did not see that the check had no signature, although every part of the check was making an impression on his eye. His brain was working too. Possibly the unconscious of the driver also had its reasons for wishing not to see that the check was imperfect. He may have been tired, or he may have had a grudge against his employer. The failure to see was purely mental. So is the failure of almost all of us purely mental when we do not see an error in a printed page. If a letter is left out we see it though it is not there. If I saw a person in my room though he was not there, we should rightly call this vision of mine an hallucination. The psychologists call the failure to see a real object a negative hallucination.

Why did I not sign the check? I was not well pleased to have my order changed from deposit account to collect on delivery. I did not intend to keep even $30.00 on deposit at Mercer's, and really did not want to take the trouble either to write to them for a check or to go in person to draw out the money. So I made a worthless check. Every mistake ever made can be explained in the same way. Every action that we do is done clearly because we have a motive for doing it, a wish to do it. Similarly every act that we omit doing has equally a wish behind it, a wish not to do that very thing.

No soldier is excused for omission of a duty because he forgot it. It is the same in love as in war. Rosalind in *As You Like It* expresses the principle that a failure to do a thing is on account of a wish not to do it, in the following words: " Break an hour's promise in love! He that will divide a minute into a thousand parts, and break but a part of the thousandth part of a minute in the affairs of love, it may be said of him that Cupid hath clapped him o' the shoulder, but I'll warrant him heart-whole."

In the case of the check unsigned, which is the case of

forgetting to write a letter of apology, or to post a letter already written, or to return a book or an umbrella, the wish is transparent enough, when once called to our attention. But it was an unconscious wish, or a wish of which we were at the time unconscious. It is the same with anyone who has " builded better than he knew." *His* unconscious has been helping him.

Another amusing mistake, which I made and which very clearly showed what I really wished to do, is as follows. I consciously wished to get up one morning at half-past six. I told my wife, who, without my knowledge, set the alarm clock for that hour. Just before I went to bed myself, I went to the alarm clock, with the conscious purpose of setting it to ring at the desired hour. I took the clock from the shelf where it was, and turned it around to see the dial where the hour of the alarm is adjusted. I saw that the indicator pointed to half-past six. So far so good. I then looked at the arm which stops the alarm bell from ringing or releases it so that it can ring at the proper time. It actually pointed to the word " alarm," but I saw only the word " silent." Unconsciously I must have made the inference that because I saw the word " silent," therefore the arm was set for silence, because what I did was to turn it. Mentally, that is consciously, at the time I thought that I was setting it for alarm, though I really turned it off, and went to bed with a perfectly satisfied conscious conscience. Next morning I slept till ten minutes of seven and awoke with a start. For twenty minutes my unconscious conscience had been trying to wake me up and had succeeded in doing so at such a time as to enable me to make, but with a great deal of hurry, the train I wished both consciously and unconsciously to catch. I certainly admire the skill of my unconscious in thus giving me a little more rest, and letting me get the train just the same. What I really wanted to do was just what I did do—namely, sleep a little longer, and catch the train too. No one will doubt that the influence of the unconscious wish which I had tried to repress was sufficient to blind me to the real positions of the mechanisms of the alarm clock. If I had been asked, just after turning it off, whether I had set the alarm, I should certainly have said I had done so, and with the clearest conscience.

In all these errors it is quite clear that there was a wish, as evident as the wish-content of Rip Van Winkle's otherwise irrelevant statement about his latest drink: ." Well, I'll not count this one." The unconscious so successfully counts out a great many things which it wills not to do or to reckon or to notice, that the things themselves simply do not occur to one's mind. And if they do not occur, what power will cause us to do those things? We may write them down, but we shall forget to look at the memorandum. We may get another person to remind us of them, but we shall either not hear him, or not listen to him, or shall reason so plausibly to ourselves why the whole thing is off anyway, that we shall feel justified, even consciously for a while, in not doing it.

A rower in a swift tide will not go directly across the stream if he goes directly across the current, but will strike the opposite shore some distance either above or below the point opposite which he started, because the current carries him up or down. If a mariner knew nothing about the Gulf Stream and attempted to steer across the ocean, he might land hundreds of miles from his purposed destination.

So in ignorance of the trend of the unconscious we do not arrive whither we aim, and we make all sorts of excuses for not doing so. But excuses or no excuses, we are forced by these blunders of ours to see that we are to a certain extent controlled by a power which is outside of our conscious life. It is not outside of our complete mental life any more than the current is outside of the river or the Gulf Stream is outside of the ocean. On the other hand, the current of the river is no more intimately a part of the river than is the unconscious a part of my mental life as a whole. If we swim in a river that has a current, and do not look at the river bank, but only at the water near us, we never know the motion of the current. We learn that we are being carried several miles an hour by the current as we swim in it only after looking at the water and the river bank at the same time. In the modern analytic psychology we have a means of seeing and estimating the influence of the mental current in which our consciousnesses are swimming. The analogy of many consciousnesses swimming in the current of one river is not so very misleading, either, as it is found that we are all carried toward the same goal by the same unconscious trend.

The importance of the new viewpoint which includes both consciousness and the unconscious is as vital as is the necessity that the navigator should allow for currents in the ocean when sailing from port to port. And as the knowledge of the modern navigator is so far advanced that the pilot of today can cross the ocean without the wastage of a mile, so the modern science of analytic psychology has superseded the older doctrine which recognized the dynamics of only the conscious mentality. For the vision into the lower strata of the mind is a deeper vision, and makes intelligible much of what was paradoxical before. For instance, it has shown what the force is, and how it operates, which controls that association of ideas, that topic which, in the mental science of the past, caused so much dispute and produced so much paradox.

Recognizing, then, the existence and the elemental power of the unconscious portion of human mentality, we are in a position to understand the simpler of its mechanisms and the effects produced by them in the outward actions and words of our fellow-beings.

Summary

The deeper knowledge of the nature of the individual, now for the first time available for teacher and parent, takes into consideration the unconscious mental activities, and a knowledge of these as they appear in the child is now an essential part of the equipment of all who hope to do the best work in the bringing up of the young. The ordinary blunder is the clearest illustration of the working of the unconscious wish.

CHAPTER II

THE UNCONSCIOUS FACTOR

As each one of us desires to develop his personality to the utmost, and as the recognition of the existence of the unconscious element in the mind as a whole at once suggests a comparison between it and the conscious element, it is a natural question to ask what kind of acts are the most personal.

What Act Is Most Personal?

Which of our acts are most likely to be regarded by ourselves as most our own? Are they those which are the most conscious or those which are the most unconscious? I think no one will hesitate to say that the acts which we perform in a state of semi-consciousness are but half ours, but what we perform with the most intense attention, what in that sense must be called the most keenly conscious acts, are those which we would be most likely to call our own. This comes to the same thing as saying that our consciousness is the most real part of us. And yet, from one point of view, our conscious life, in which we seem to take the greatest amount of interest, is the smallest part of our mental life. I dismiss for the moment the question of being able to call by the name mental what is not conscious. Modern psychology goes on the principle that it is, and that no proper and complete account can be given of the whole mental life which does not give acknowledgment to the unconscious.

But there we have what seems to be a dilemma. What is most important is what is most proper to the ego, and what is most peculiarly the ego's is consciousness. But when compared to the extent and the depth of the unconscious part of the mind, the conscious part seems most unimportant. The truth is that the two parts have different rôles in the drama of life, and that life would be incomplete, at least human life would, without both of them. Not only does the unconscious mental life play a great rôle in the adjustments which are necessarily made between the physical organism and the complexities of modern life, in causing adaptations, of which we are never conscious, of the various physiological functions to the ever changing environment of the life of today, but the unconscious wishes are forever causing mental, and purely mental, *not* physiological, changes to take place in our minds, of whose results only and not the processes we are conscious.

Not only do we eat new and unaccustomed foods, to which our unconscious powers are obliged to adjust our digestive apparatus, but we are fed from time to time upon new and unaccustomed mental pabulum which requires a change in our attitude towards many things. In these days we are gradually adapting ourselves mentally to the mental atmosphere of a nation at war. The sight of multitudes of uniformed men, which would in previous years have been extremely exciting to all of us, is *now* seen with quite another feeling, which has been produced in us by a great many circumstances to which we do not consciously attend, and yet there is a change, and a great one, which has taken place, in our hearts we call it in common parlance. The sight of women running trolley cars and elevators and acting as ticket choppers on street railway systems, although we do not make much conscious comment on it, is nevertheless a factor in the total change which is being wrought in our unconscious mentality.

We Are Most What We Most Desire

In one sense what we call most our own spiritually is what we have consciously desired most and most earnestly striven to secure the attainment of. But there are in each one of us a great many desires, and strong ones too, of which we are totally unconscious. When, after a certain amount of study of the newer wish psychology, we come to realize how great and how strong these unconscious desires are, we for a time begin to think that those are really the most peculiarly our own and in a sense ourselves, our real selves. Frequently what we have consciously most desired we find after its attainment giving us comparatively little or no pleasure. We cease to want many things, such as riches, when once we have got them.

If what we most desire is what we ourselves most are, then the converse of this proposition is that our desires most exactly represent us. 'Now, if this is true and if it is also true that the greater number of our desires are absolutely unknown to us, then the conclusion naturally follows that of ourselves we know comparatively little. It is only the superficial conscious desires that we really know, and we are all frequently puzzled by their apparent contradictions, not to say by the manifest inability of some persons to form any idea of why they want this or that thing. The phenomenon of the capricious will is quite familiar in the case of children. They are expected to wish this and that and to be unable to say why. The modern form of psychology, sometimes called the wish psychology, has given an answer to many of these problems. Its answer is that all the unconscious wishes are forms of the creative wish for reproduction, and that the reason why they have been forced into unconsciousness is that things sexual have been tabooed in many civilizations. The fact that these desires have been forced into unconsciousness accounts for the fact that they never enter consciousness except under disguise. For instance, it has been repeatedly shown that among many others the unduly strong desire to smoke tobacco or to use certain kinds of foods is a compensation for certain wishes for the more direct form of physical creativeness against which society has set up a strong barrier, and the unconscious, groping like a blind animal, or stretching forth like a blade of grass under a board toward the light, takes, in its struggle, an indirect way towards gratification instead of the most direct which has been blocked.

From the multitudinous prohibitions aimed by society at the exploitation of things directly sexual has come a sort of idea, partly conscious and partly unconscious in the minds of men and women alike, that such things are wicked or sinful or at least dangerous. It is called playing with fire, with the implication that all those who play with fire are likely to be burned, furthermore that it is a bad thing in every way to be burned. A state of society is conceivable in which such a fear of being burned did not exist and in which therefore there would be plenty of

people in evidence who had been burned and been dis-
figured by their burns.   Now, the fact is that in avoiding
the one kind of burns we are suffering another kind.
What we are really doing is exchanging a physical for a
mental burn.   There is an absolute law of the conserva-
tion of energy in the mental as well as in the physical
world.   What we gain in the way of physical advantage
by our constant curbing of the natural instincts, which is
the name which we have given to the primordial urge
toward the maintenance of the individual and of the race,
is lost in mental advantage.   For the absolutely natural
and therefore wholesome instinct of the girl to be a
mother is constantly being repressed and in our present
civilization is in many cases not being replaced in any
way by a socially valuable substitute.

There is nothing to which one can devote his or her
whole heart, to use the common expression, which does
not enlist all the instincts with which nature has so generously provided us; there is, in short, no activity available
for us that will not leave some of the instinctive desire
ungratified, unless it enlists the whole of our personality,
including the unconscious wishes above referred to.   In
other words, unless we can find something to do which
satisfies our conscious desires, which we have seen above
to be at best whimsical and illogical, and at the same time
gratifies in some substitutive form the unconscious wishes,
which are a very great proportion of the motive force of
all human action, we shall not be working, or playing
either for that matter, with our entire available energy,
and therefore we shall be working at cross-purposes with
ourselves.

The unconscious wishes, even if they are not known

and taken into account, are nevertheless wishes, just as strong as the conscious ones if not much stronger, and are operative in our bodies even if they are quite outside of our ken. The net result in many instances is their counteracting the energy of the conscious wishes, and nullifying the effect of the latter. That is the explanation of why a great many good things go wrong, and a great many otherwise good men too.

Therefore, we can return to our first question as to what kind of deeds are the most personal. If it is a matter of mathematical proportion, such that we could say that the wishes having the greatest strength or the greatest number best represented the personality of the individual, we should be in a position to say that the most conscious acts, or those which we feel most consciously desirous of performing, are the least our own. They are the fewest in number and the weakest in dynamics. On the other hand, the unconscious wishes, those indeed which the conscious personality is constantly striving to repress, are the ones which most exactly represent what we really are. Now, if this is the case, as a great many modern psychologists firmly believe, and if we therefore really know the smallest part of our true nature, it would seem to be a great advantage if we should be so trained as to be able to learn about these unconscious wishes and learn, too, to be able to control them to our own advantage and profit. Our present-day education gives us not an inkling of this dual nature of our everyday mind. Only a few advanced scientists have taken it into consideration. Some men have instinctively gained a control over themselves and united their unconscious and their conscious selves, but the majority of humans, no matter how speciously civilized and conventional they may be, have failed of the spiritual union within themselves which is so rare a thing.

A curious and interesting corollary to the principle that we do not ourselves understand our dual nature is that while the real Mr. A does not thoroughly understand himself, although he thinks he does, Mr. B unconsciously appreciates and measures both the conscious and the unconscious Mr. A and acts accordingly. The folly of others is perfectly patent to everybody. This folly is the result of the split between the conscious wishes and the unconscious.

Continuous Unconscious Estimation

One cannot avoid thinking that the unconscious is continually estimating the value, according to its primeval standards, of its entire environment. A machine, without so-called human intelligence, would do the same thing, if it was furnished with the delicate apparatus which is found in the human organism. If we but suppose it to contain but the feeling of liking and dislike, and the tendency to promote the things that cause the liking and reject those which cause the feeling of dislike, we shall have the medium for the expression of a great deal of action which looks like human intelligence. Every situation will, in itself, contain the factors whose product will be a plus or minus balance with regard to the desirability or undesirability of its continuance. If we suppose that the situation as a whole includes not only the actual material physical surroundings of the individual, in so far as he can sense them, but also the factor contributed by the physiological nature of the human body, we shall have all that is necessary to account for the variability of the valuations of human experience.   For the same external situation will evoke now one and now another reaction; it will be desired or it will be disliked not because of any inherent quality in itself but because of a difference of the state of the physical organism of the body.

If that is the case, we must infer that the unconscious, which is the sum total of the reactions to the environment, or to the particular situation in which the body finds itself from moment to moment, is constantly producing tensions for or against different factors in the situation, and that we, as consciousnesses, are quite unaware of those tensions.   If we meet a person for the first time, and shake hands and pass a few remarks about the weather or the war, it is unthinkable that the physical organism, both of ourselves and of the person we meet, is not responding to sensations of sight, sound, touch, temperature, odour—in fact, every quality which *could,* and even those which could not, be perceived, if the conscious attention were directed to them.   Although we had formed only a dim idea of dislike for the person we casually met, and though we might later be advised that he was not personally clean, and that an odour of perspiration was perceptible about him, we could realize that we had ourselves dimly perceived that odour, and believe it quite likely that we had formed a dislike for him on that account alone.   Also while in his presence, if some third person had called to our attention that the person to whom we were being introduced did not look us squarely in the eye, but had a furtive glance, we could then consciously note this characteristic, although, without this hint from the third person, we might have utterly failed to notice it.

In other words, observation of small details like those just mentioned, while it may not be conscious, is inevitably made by the unconscious part of the mind, and is made all the time, and includes every detail of every situation in which we find ourselves. The proof is that we frequently recall characteristics of persons and things after we have ceased to have them as a part of our immediate situation, and we notice retrospectively that they were thus and so. Later conscious observation confirms the facts. Therefore we must suppose that, while conscious observation is very limited in extent, unless one is trained in it for some purpose, like the magician Houdin, the observations which we make upon persons and things are made and completely made, and with no effort on our part,—they are automatically registered as are the details on a photographic film, but they do not enter consciousness. Of course it is a great economy that this should be the case. It would be a great waste of time for us consciously to make a catalogue of all the phases of the appearance and actions of every chance person we met and every scene we passed through. But it is quite certain that this is being done in us by our unconscious all the time, and that only the net results of this unconscious observation are occasionally sent up into consciousness. In their place, below the threshold of consciousness, these observations and records are of great value, as they enable us to form intuitive judgments, as they are called, which generally come as near to being correct as we can consciously make.*

* Cf. what is said (p. 33 ff.) about unconscious inference.

Primeval Standards

I said that the unconscious is making judgments according to primeval standards. A study of the unconscious, carried on now for nearly a quarter of a century according to psychoanalytical methods, has established the fact that, as we go down deeper into the strata of the unconscious, we find simpler and more elemental activities. The unconscious is primarily concerned with hunger and sex. Without the barriers which society, even the most barbarous, has set up against the unlicensed gratification of these two cravings, the individual would at once, and every time in every situation, proceed to the satisfaction of both needs. It is repulsive to many people to think that the attraction which other people have for them, and they themselves for the others, is solely and merely a crass sexual one at bottom. But if it is a fact, why blink it? It would horrify some pretty young woman school teacher to be told that the influence of her personality was due primarily to her physically sexual charms. It would seem to vitiate all of the ideals which she had held before her of spiritual and intellectual superiority. Does she think that her influence over the boys of her class is merely due to her mental cleverness? Do I seem cynical in making these remarks? If it can be shown to be a fact, does it really spoil the whole relation between her and her boy pupils? If it could be demonstrated to her beyond possibility of doubt that her attraction of girls was a homosexual one, would that necessarily make her an undesirable teacher? I think not. But I think that her knowledge of these fundamental facts will be of service to her in improving the quality of her relation between herself and the pupils of both sexes.

A teacher *should* know the tools with which he or she is working, and *all* the means of producing an effect on his pupils, and this one of unconscious emotions, or as we might call them, to make them more comprehensible, unconscious causes for attraction and repulsion, is one of the most important questions which comes up in the schoolroom. It is the dynamo which supplies all the power for all the machinery in the schoolroom workshop. To ignore it is folly. To learn all about it that can be learned is the nearest approach that can be made to wisdom.

The Unconscious Factor (a Specific Instance)

When the mind is most concentrated upon some one thing, say a column of figures which one is adding, there are elements in the very object of the keenest attention which entirely escape attention—of which the mind is totally unconscious. There is a man adding a column of figures. Outwardly he is insensible of everything, does not know that the weather is hot, that he is physically uncomfortable, sitting on a hard seat in a strained position, reading his figures with tired eyes and in an insufficent light. He adds the tens and units of each

17
83
52
69
84
43
68
———
416

number alternately, from the top downward, saying to himself as he does so: 17, 20, 100, 102, 152, 161, 221, 225, 305, 308, 348, 351, 411; and then verifies by taking the numbers upward, saying: 68, 71, 111, 115, 195, 204, 264, 266, 316, 319, 399, 416. It does not agree with the first time, and finally he finds that in going downward he has said 351 for 356, having repeated the 3 of 43 (next to last number) instead of saying the 8 of 68. Of the numbers alone he was aware. But what made him take the 3 instead of the 8? That was taking the 3 twice. Had he any special predilection for threes? He had. Everyone has, for it is the number which has, in the hinterland of the mind, the closest connection with creativeness, and everyone would be creative. Also the number ignored is 5. The number 5 is linked in the memory of the race with weakness and solitude. Hence it tends to be expunged or forgotten in favour of 3, wherever there is a possible alternative between them as here. Would this indicate that mistakes of dropping fives are more common than the other errors? Surely they are, when fives are rivals of threes in operations involving unconscious mentality.

This is a case which I took as an example of the most vivid consciousness. The person adding was supremely conscious of figures. His whole attention was occupied by figures to the exclusion of every other thought and sensation. If one spoke to him, he would not hear, until after he had satisfied himself that his addition was correct. Then either of two things might happen. He might suddenly become conscious that he *had been* spoken to, and say: " Oh, did you speak? ", or he might have been conscious of being spoken to, but voluntarily ignored it, till he was through, and then replied to the remark.

However it may be, we have him in an intensely conscious state, possibly better described as intensively conscious. But even in that state we find him absolutely unconscious, for the time, of the error he has made. He is unconscious not merely of the physical conditions of his body, but he is unconscious of a part of the very thing that he is most conscious of. It may seem a platitude to say that one is naturally unconscious of mistakes while one is making them. Of course, every error is an unwitting one, else it would be not an error but a voluntary perversion or diversion. But why are some wrong actions errors and others perversions? Why are they not all voluntary perversions? Do we not want, all of us, to do what is right, and are we not, all of us, awake, especially when we are doing additions? From this it appears that one is likely to have unconscious states of mind peppered through the most conscious states. When the man said 351 where he should have said 356 in order to be correct, he was fully conscious of saying 351, but he was not aware that 351 was not correct.

We might say that he was fully awake to the number, but asleep to its incorrectness. Thus it appears that one is awake to a thing, that is, a sensation or a thought, but asleep to the relation of the thought and the thing. We have here, then, come upon a general rule, namely that things (sensations, thoughts) are more easily objects of consciousness than relations are. One can be perfectly awake to a thing and absolutely anaesthetic to many of its relations.

But there is more to it than that. The man adding the column of figures was wide awake to something that did not exist. He was conscious of something that was not there. He created it out of nothing. Didn't create anything? Only said 351? But where did the 351 come from? It was formed from the combination of things already in his mind. But it came from the repetition of a 3 instead of the addition of an 8. How could that happen? It happened in spite of the presence of the 8. The 8 was ignored. The man shut his eyes to it, so to speak. The

3 supervened and obliterated the 8. So the prime question is about where the 3 came from. That has been hinted at above in saying that in the unconscious life of the race the number 3 is associated with creativeness. For we can easily understand that if there is a general tendency, such as creativeness, which is going to make itself felt, to push itself forward whenever it can, and add its colour, as it were, to every expression of thought, it will always be present in every thought in whatever strength it can.

If, for instance, there is a word which we are seeking in our minds, we may say that our mind has in it at the time a hole of a certain shape, which can be filled with only the right word. Every other word will be a misfit. Now if there should be two words which fit the hole, and one of these words is more associated with the general trends of the unconscious than the other, it will naturally be supplied first. That amounts to saying that, in the selection of words while we are composing, we are governed by the principle of the line of least resistance, in thought, just as in physics. It is about the same, too, as saying that in thought, and in this matter of the choice of synonyms in particular, the actual word selected is the algebraic sum of all the forces that are possessed by each and every word that may have any claim at all to come into consciousness in connection with the theme on which we are writing. The same thing takes place in adding a column of figures. We are apt to regard the different digits as having no peculiarities of their own, but that is not the case. Every number, and particularly the smaller numbers, has an individuality of its own. It is itself a little centre of force, a force which it has acquired through the ages of human thinking, and when there is a balance between the one number and the other as was the case in the addition above mentioned, the number which is the stronger will come up into consciousness and replace the weaker number. It seems quite extraordinary to regard an absolutely impersonal number, a mere counter, as having a force of its own, but that is exactly what I mean to say it has, if we look upon it not as merely a written or printed word or figure, but a state of mind, as in the illustration above given it undeniably is.

When we realize that so elementary a thing as a digit or a single word is a centre of force, it becomes much easier to understand that other mental activities are also forces and that the net result of their operation, as we see it in a sentence or a paragraph or a book, is a highly complex result, which only the most thoroughgoing analysis can reduce to its elements. And if a book, a novel, a play or a system of philosophy is the algebraic sum of all the forces operating in the mind of the writer it is equally true that all other expressions of individuality, all conduct and every individual act, are quite as much the effects of all the causes, both mental and physical, which have preceded it.

These forces we group under the name of wishes. The force of the conscious wish is quite familiar to everyone. A person, that is, a normal person, wishing for a thing, goes right along on the best known path of acquirement and keeps going until he gets it. The contribution of the newer psychology to this subject is that it is not merely the conscious wishes whose fulfilment one is seeking from hour to hour and from minute to minute, but that there is a far larger number of unconscious wishes which are inexorably driving us to do things all the time, big things, little things and medium things.   One can satisfy a conscious and an unconscious wish both at the same time.   This is shown by the sum in addition, where the correct sum was what was consciously desired, and the mistake was a partial satisfaction of an unconscious wish for creativeness.   In fact every error of any kind whatever, whether a mistake in addition, a slip of the tongue or of the pen, a faulty memory or a wrong act of reasoning, an erroneously carried out action or a course of conduct based on a carefully reasoned plan, are one and all the expressions of wishes, partly conscious, partly unconscious.*

That one can satisfy a conscious and an unconscious wish at one and the same time is shown very clearly by the choice of words in writing.   It is quite evident in the composition of a poem, where not only is each word the satisfaction of a wish, but every thought, every figure of speech, every mind picture which is evoked in the mind of the poet and afterward in his readers' minds.   The most popular pieces of literature are those which most gratify the wishes of the readers, and to a large extent the unconscious wishes.   I have shown that in my analysis of the figure of onomatopoeia on page 108.   The wish gratified by imitative language is an unconscious one. When I recite to my classes the Greek line given on page 108, and also that where Chryseis steps from the boat,

Εκ δη Χρυσηις νηος βη ποντοποροιο,
'Ek de | 'Chryse | 'is ne | 'os be | 'pontopo | 'roio

the hearers even though they know no Greek are amused by the similarity   f the rhythm of the words to the rhythm

* See pages 167 and 257.

of the actions of the girl, but they are quite unconscious of what wish is there satisfied. Also lines like that of Tennyson quoted in the same section are liked because of the same quality. But the hearers do not know why they like them. They are just nice, or beautiful, or pretty, or grand, as the case may be, and that is as far as the analysis of the hearer goes, and it is as far as it is necessary for it to go, in most cases.

But when it comes to making mistakes which involve an injury or a loss of money or life, then it becomes important to know the true causes. Likewise when it is found that some men and women can turn out a far greater amount of work than others, it becomes interesting if not important, and it surely is important in these times of war, to find out the exact cause of these differences in the efficiency of different people. To that end many elaborate experiments have been made and are being made daily, but enough attention has not yet been given to the causes which lie in the unconscious lives of the workers.

In the schoolroom every mistake will take on a new interest for the teacher, when it is realized that it comes not from any faulty construction in the brains of the pupils but (in the majority of cases) from adverse desire on the part of the child, a desire of which the child is generally utterly unaware, and which, when the newer psychology has permeated through the schools, will be controlled to the great advantage both of the individual pupil and of the country as a whole. It is the teachers, too, who will be the ones with the greatest opportunity of remedying the defects inherent in present-day education by bringing to their task a knowledge of the unconscious working of the mind. In the schoolroom there is the opportunity to a slight extent, and later I trust there will be a greater time given for the purpose, to analyse the minds of as many children who need it as possible. Of course it is needed only in the pupils who are doing unsatisfactory work. The others do not require the same study. But it will be found that those children who have the greatest difficulty in doing their lessons are those in whom there is the greatest number of unconscious wishes going against the successful accomplishment of their work.

And this brings me again to the theme of the fulfilment simultaneously of both unconscious and conscious wishes. For it is a safe assumption that many if not all of those who do poor work would like to do good work, if only to gain the glory which comes from any kind of achievement. But analysis of every situation where bad work is done reveals an unconscious wish on the part of the pupil to do bad work. There is in the defectiveness of the work a satisfaction gained by the defective worker. Either it is an amount of sympathy from some parent, or a wish, of which also the child may be entirely unconscious, to " get back at " somebody with poor work. Possibly a parent has untactfully commanded the child to accomplish some school task, and the unconscious antagonism, natural to every man, woman or child, against authority is thereby aroused; possibly the task is rejected by the child on account of some real or fancied sickness, as Tom Tulliver, in *The Mill on the Floss,* said it gave him a toothache, the only sickness he ever had, to study Euclid.

There are thus always more wishes than one satisfied in every act, in all conduct. Unhappiness always results where the unconscious wish, operating against conscious ones, which are those imposed upon the individual by society, is fulfilled; and the happiness which sometimes is found, as by the boy who plays truant and goes fishing or swimming, is never without the element of unhappiness caused by the conflict with society.

So that every mistake in addition or in any mathematical or other work in school is the result of two kinds of wishes operating in conjunction yet in opposition. The strongest *has* to win. The problem for the teacher is to strengthen the conscious wishes by aligning the unconscious wishes with them, by reinforcing them with the unconscious wishes. It can be done, and it is being done, but with less success than if the knowledge of the existence of the unconscious wish were a perfectly conscious knowledge. I call it an imperfectly conscious knowledge of human motives, and a partly unconscious knowledge of them, to go on the general principle that emulation and ambition and desire for mastery and for praise is likely to make boys or girls do their best. It is really necessary for the teacher and the parent to find out why sometimes these appeals to well-known motives do not have on the pupils or offspring the effects which they are supposed to have.

If it is taken into consideration how complex are the mental processes of even the youngest children, and how strong an unconscious desire may be, and how every act is the satisfaction of both conscious and unconscious desires at the same time, it may be possible to find in each case which is studied with care the unconscious element which is spoiling the whole product. In a glass manufactory a certain amount of glass turned out was of an inferior quality because its colour was not right. The manager told the owner that one of the hands had thrown a screwdriver into the mechanical mixer and that the relative strength of one of the components, soda, had been changed thereby. It was found by the owner, when he examined the machinery, that no such thing had happened. The manager had through an oversight, which he was ashamed to confess, allowed the tank supplying the soda to the mixer to become empty. Now, I believe that teachers, as a whole, are too conscientious to allow the failure of any ingredients which they know about. They are quite as careful and competent as the owners (parents) in this case. But the point is that the ingredient necessary to make a high order of academic glass in this simile is generally unknown both to the owner and the manager alike. In this case, through ignorance of properties it might have in turning out a thoroughly perfect product, the soda is not used at all.

Marion Crawford's *Marietta* contains the story of the secret ingredient which gave to medieval Venetian glass its wonderful colour. Now, the wonderful quality of *some* of the natural product of the human mind is due to an ingredient, so to speak, that has been sought for through the ages. It is the aim of educators to make a product which shall be equal to the best natural product; in other words, to train *all* persons to be nearly as possible the spiritual and intellectual equals of those great men and women who have had no education, or who, having the same education as their very inferior coevals, have distinguished themselves by being in every way superior to their contemporaries.

Just as the colour and other qualities of glass are due to the ingredients and to the manner of handling them, so it is clear that there is in the mind a constant stream of what we might call ingredients, in the shape of wishes or trends or tendencies, the sum of all of which inevitably makes up the final product that enters consciousness. Most educational theory up to the present has been based on the hypothesis that all the ingredients were conscious ones. Educational treatises, to be sure, have chapters on the instincts, and on habit and other topics, but the treatment of any of these topics which leaves out any consideration of the unconscious tendencies is sure to be incomplete and misleading. To describe the mind without the unconscious factor is to rehearse *Hamlet* without the Prince of Denmark, a mere rehearsal, and no true performance.

Unconscious Inference

" The spirit is willing, but the flesh is weak " might be applied to the so-called inability of the pupil to grasp certain propositions and the relation between them. Take, for instance, in arithmetic the circumstance that some children cannot remember the multiplication table or have difficulty in remembering it. We may think that their spirit is willing, and their natural ability small, but there is very little difference in the natural retentiveness of individual minds. The difference in the ability to remember six times seven equals forty-two is a difference in willingness to accept, not the truth of the statement but the statement itself, in the first place. The attempt on the part of the teacher to evoke this numerical relation through the reasoning powers of the child is quite as likely to arouse his natural unconscious antagonism as is the imperious demand that he shall memorize the whole table of 6s. Both of them make an appeal to him to do something that he cannot see the use of doing. In the proposition that

$6 \times 1 = 6$ he has no interest because it is so flatly self-evident that it seems sheer nonsense to waste time about it. With the other multiples of 6 he has no concern unless the numbers can symbolize something to him, as, for instance, that $6 \times 2 = 12$ looks like the shape, now current, of a box of eggs holding a dozen. The trouble is that he cannot *do* anything with these facts. They will not propel a coaster or tease a girl, or anything else interesting. His flesh is strong enough, meaning the plasticity of his brain tissue, but his spirit is unwilling. There is indeed nothing in the nature of the multiplication table itself which should make his spirit willing. It is only some association that can be made with it that will show him that he can do things with it that will make him want to use it. The same is true of most of the subjects of study.

Frequently in academic studies one comes upon some proposition from which it is necessary to abstract and derive the elements and make a catalogue of all the possible permutations of the combinations of these elements, before one can truly be said to understand the subject. While this mechanical method of thought is natural to any highly organized machine such as is the human mind, it is in the latter buried deep in the unconscious, and it is difficult for all children and for most adults to evoke it.

The various versions of the two propositions which head this section, about the spirit being willing but the flesh being weak, would be quite as uninteresting to the average adult as are the multiple combinations of numbers to the average child. Just as the child cannot see what he can *do* with six times four equals twenty-four, so the average adult has not yet been able to see what he can do with the different forms in which the same proposition can be cast. The versions, which are carefully catalogued in formal logic, with rules about which of them may and may not be inferred from each of the others are already formed in the unconscious, and they operate there in such a way as to produce in some individuals some strange inhibitions. The rules of formal logic are the work of the conscious mind, and they are dry and mechanical enough. They might also be called the development of the unconscious thought which is behind all correct conscious reasoning, and, when we think, we ought to get clear and logical results, but we do not, for the unconscious wish continually selects the one which is most consistent with it, regardless of scientific truth.

When a child tells a lie, the cause of his action in telling it is one that exists in his unconscious wish. The rules of formal logic apply only to the impartial development of all the thoughts, and not to the selection of one of them. Formal logic takes cognizance only of the verbal form in which a statement is made and not why the individual makes that statement, and the numerous statements that might be made are all in logical form, but are selected only on a basis of their congruence with the unconscious wish.

The cause of most persons' making any statement is generally that they wish it were true, and the louder they affirm it, or the more eloquently they can ring the changes on the same wish expressed in various ways, the more do they seem (to themselves) to get a fulfilment of that wish. But they do not see or in any way become cognizant of the latent wish. They do not realize that the satisfaction they get out of making that statement emphatically and in various forms is a satisfaction of the wish that it might be a true statement. There is even a real satisfaction in proclaiming that a subject, say Latin, is hard. What is the total situation, if it really is hard? First, those who do not succeed in learning it well, have what comfort they may derive from the fact that too hard a subject has been given them for any except the phenomenally brilliant pupil. Those who do succeed in it have a very solid sense of superiority which is of course very wholesome and beneficial and gives them the confidence to attack other subjects which may be harder. But the reiterated statement of a child that any task is hard is only the conscious expression of an unconscious wish to have it difficult, either so difficult that it is impossible, or difficult enough either to excuse bad performance or bring generous reward of praise for a good one. Similarly of any vehement statement whatever, as that Emily cheated or Tom has had more of the teacher's attention or good will, and therefore took a higher rank than he deserved, or what not. The obvious advantages to the accuser, if the statements were true, are a matter quite apart from formal logic, which would have to employ the cumbrous syllogism to prove it, but are evidently an unmistakable expression of an unconscious wish to be relieved of a responsibility which would cause in the child a sense of inferiority if the responsibility were not rejected.

The same holds true of all adults' statements. The assertion that a criminal is wholly bad is necessary to justify his being executed or jailed for life, and, if we have disposed of him in either of these ways, we can but wish it were true, or, as we express it, hope that it is true, because if it is not true, we are ourselves in the very unenviable position of committing a wrong quite as inexcusable as the criminal's. If on the contrary we declare that any person or thing is absolutely good, we are but expressing our desire to have him (or her or it) quite perfect. And when we proclaim a person or thing as superlatively excellent we are asserting at the same time our own excellence in being able to see and point out the excellent qualities. All of which is quite apart from logic. It is, on the other hand, psycho-logic, which literally means only the *words of the spirit* (the soul, which is complete and unified longing, asserting itself in words).

The unconscious is continually working out the permutations mentioned above and, for the purpose of rationalization, is delivering statements for acceptance by the conscious mind, that are exactly these versions of the original statement, which is the true one. But the contradictory is the one offered by the unconscious and accepted by the conscious mind. The acceptability of the contradictory, " The spirit is willing, but the flesh is weak," is partly conditioned by the fact that as a proposition it is in perfect form. It has a form, indeed, which is quite as flawless as the others. The only difference in form is that in the word weak there is an implied negative, because it means " not strong."

The Psychological Negative

The force of the negative in unconscious thinking is virtually *nil*. There is no such thing as a psychological negative. The verbal negation of an idea is that idea unchanged, save for the verbal addition of the word " not," which has no psychological value whatever. To tell a child not to do what it is doing is equivalent to saying: " I see you are doing that. I congratulate you on your ability to do it. And you are doing it against the strong opposition of my will, which shows that you are strong yourself, even stronger than I am, particularly if you can go on doing it in opposition to my will." The only way to abolish an idea or stop an action is to replace it with another idea. Then the first idea disappears and is negatived in the only way possible. It is supremely difficult for some teachers (parents, or average business men, too, for that matter) to abolish the idea from their own consciousness. It takes hold of them, by virtue of the very dynamic quality it receives from the fact that it implies a struggle of wills. There is no value to such a struggle of wills. If the teacher's will prevails, there is a defeat to that of the pupil and one of the chief ends of education, the development of will on the part of the pupil, has been frustrated. The teacher, strong before, has been strengthened, and the pupil, weak before, has been weakened, and has had initiated in his soul, if not confirmed, the habit of giving in, which, existing in some of the best trained children, is a continual impediment to their success in after life. Success in later life depends upon the habit of conquering. So that when a situation arises in which there presents itself an opportunity for the battle of wills between teacher and pupil (parent and child, businessman and employee) the quality of the future performance of pupil, child or employee is detrimentally affected. It is much better not to have a conflict of personal wills, and particularly in the school. It may be of remote possible benefit in the home, but I doubt it. It may be of great advantage occasionally in business, but that does not so much concern us here. In the school, when a teacher thinks it necessary to say " Don't," let him or her weigh carefully the possibilities of avoiding a struggle of wills which will result only to the detriment of the pupil. If there is to be any conquering on the part of the pupil, and I believe that the whole school life of the child ought to be one continuous victory, that victory should be, for obvious reasons, not one over the teacher, but over the work which is being superintended by the teacher. A habit of victory should indeed be developed in the child even if it is necessary to include a victory over the teacher, and over the school rules, in order best to develop the willpower of the child; but the essential point is missed entirely if the battle rages between the pupil and the teacher. If it is inevitable that that must occur, it is better for the pupil to conquer. I know that it is well for a person to know when he is beaten, and that it is a good thing to learn to accept defeat gracefully, but a training in the acceptance of defeat is not a good training for a child to fit him for competition in the external world of life.

So it is of the utmost importance, for teacher and pupil as well, to devote their mental and physical activities to the accomplishment of the academic tasks. The personal relation of superiority or inferiority in point of willpower comes up again and again in the schoolroom as everywhere else. It has a tendency to come up, simply because of the fact that the teacher is human as well as the child, and that the fundamental desire of the unconscious of every human is to be superior. In this connection we may clearly see the great disadvantage which it sometimes is for a child, particularly a boy, to have a very strong-willed father. The domination of the father produces a habit of servility in the child which he tends to evince in his relations with all persons with whom he comes in contact in later life. If such a child comes in school in contact with a teacher of strongly domineering character, a character which, by the way, is fostered in teachers by the very atmosphere of any school, he will get no training which will offset the very adverse conditions of his home life. It would be better for such a child to be sent to a school where the teachers had been trained to allow the children themselves to domineer. In such a school the bashful, doubtful, quelled spirit might learn something of the habit of mastery.

But of course the thing cannot be done that way. The teacher must recognize that the most vital purpose of the academic education is to train the pupil to master his physical environment, so far as that can be done without interfering with the equal development of mastery in the other pupils. The tendency will always be to develop along the line of mastery of persons and not things, and this, too, has its great value, but it seems to me that in school the struggle should be directed to the mastery of things and not persons. Because of the unconscious tendency to turn the attention to persons and away from things, and this on the part of pupil and teacher alike, this sticking to the point in academic education is a very difficult matter.

To return to the consideration of the unconscious permutations of propositions—for instance, that the spirit is willing. This is the contradictory of the proposition that the spirit is unwilling, and the flesh is weak is the contradictory of the flesh is strong. Thus by the introduction of the negative word we have four propositions:

1. The spirit is willing and the flesh is strong.
2. The spirit is willing, but the flesh is weak.
3. The spirit is unwilling, but the flesh is strong.
4. The spirit is unwilling and the flesh is weak.

The second or biblical form of these statements (uttered as a truth acceptable to consciousness, because it is a palliation of circumstances, and therefore an assertion of superiority) is a transformation of the truth which is expressed in the first: The spirit is willing and the flesh is strong. This last arrangement of the ideas represents the gist of the teaching of psychoanalysis. The doctrine of the unconscious teaches too that all these permutations are in the unconscious, ready for selection. The assertion of the weakness of the child's flesh is an assertion of the superiority of the teacher. If the child's spirit is willing and his flesh is strong, and the results of education are as meagre as they are today, then the teacher feels that he is somehow to blame.

With strong flesh and willing spirit each individual ought to be perfect. I will not mention the teachers who think that both the spirit is unwilling and the flesh is weak. But the teacher feels less responsible if he can say that the flesh is weak. The child that does not make a good showing cannot do so, even with the help of the teacher, and no one is to blame.

No. 3—the spirit is unwilling and the flesh is strong— is the unconscious attitude of the child toward school work, and he is not to blame for it. Neither are the teachers nor for that matter is anyone else. It is in this as it has been in the case of other scientific advance. Wireless telegraphy and aeronautics are examples of the present condition of the practical applications of physical science. In mental science we are as far back as the days of stage coaches and pony post. The discovery of the uses to which a knowledge of the unconscious may be put is about on the same level of development as the knowledge gained by the immediate successors of Benjamin Franklin concerning the nature and use of electricity. We have, in a sense, got the unconscious on a wire, but we have not yet been able to transmute it into power with the same success that has been attained by the mechanical devices which are transforming Niagara into light, power and transportation.

In making the list of permutations of the willing spirit and strong flesh ideas we have been bringing into consciousness (a dreary task, I hear some say) what was implicitly worked out in the unconscious and is worked out not only with that but with every other possible proposition that could be made with words or even without words and merely with situations. Words are only the imperfect translations of situations into verbal form. What is to tiresome about the mere bringing of these permutations into consciousness is the fact that we have not yet grasped the bearing of these particular concrete mechanisms of thought, which are combinations of two ideas and a negative word, upon human conduct and especially that part of human conduct constituted by words themselves. But the unconscious is like a machine which can take any proposition and combine it with any other, affirmatively or negatively. From all these permutations that one is selected which is least objectionable to the Censor.* And our attitude toward education is largely that of proposition No. 2: The spirit is willing, but the flesh is weak. We think that the pupil wants to learn, that he is willing to do the tasks we set before him, but we have really failed to see that while his conscious spirit is willing, his unconscious is not, and that the unconscious part of him is by far the larger and stronger.

Also we have failed to realize that the language of the unconscious is acts *and* words, acts forming as great an amount of its language, in proportion to words, as is the general ratio of the unconscious to the conscious. The acts of all children are almost all unconscious. In the rarest cases do children really know what they are doing, and in many adults we find an almost complete ignorance of what is the true significance of a very large proportion of what they are doing from hour to hour. Particularly significant too is what we are not doing. Taken together, what one does and what one avoids doing constitute a perfect picture of one's character. Now, that perfect picture is constantly before the unconscious of every observer, and this huge mirror so to speak reflects, to those who dare look in it, exactly what our real character is. Or regarded as an enormous computing instrument, the unconscious hands us out the sum of the product or the remainder or the quotient (all being the results of the unconscious computation), and we have not an idea of how the machine did its work, any more than the average person has a clear idea of how comptometers work or what to do with them when they do not work well.

* Cf. pages 50 and 107.

But the teacher should not be the average person. He should not, though he does, see as little into the working of the mind of the child as does the average person see into the mechanics of the adding machine. To carry this simile a little farther, the teacher, up to date, has been required to know little more about the inner workings of the comptometers that he has before him in groups of ten to sixty, according to circumstances, than he would have if he only brushed off the dust with a rag and sat down before each one and worked it madly for a minute at a time, and then rushed at the next one and hammered it for another minute, and so on, and did the same sum on them all, marked the wrong ones failures and put them in another room to see if the air in that room would not improve their accuracy.

As teachers, however, we should know the intimate workings of the rods, bearings, pawls, ratchets, springs, type-bars, ribbons, etc., of every human comptometer which we have in our classes. We are not fulfilling our highest function, which, to be sure, no board of education ever requires of us, if we do not learn as much as we can of the thought mechanisms, conscious *and* unconscious. Our sole duty is not to exercise the machines and limber them up, much as some automobiles have to be towed " in speed " to get them to go themselves. That may be a very great service, but my thesis is that the human mechanisms which are driven in shoals into our classrooms are almost all out of repair; and merely to turn the wheels of a machine which is not in order is as bad as trying to crank a gas engine without turning on the spark. And under the sleek hood of each school child, and behind all their radiators (of various designs), is an engine of which many teachers wrongly believe they are merely the drivers, and not required to understand how the engine, when out of order, may be repaired.

But if we realized that when some such statement as that the spirit is willing but the flesh is weak is the reverse of truth, and that we can progress with that as a motive power about as fast as an automobile moves forward when the speed-change lever is in " reverse," we should be most eager to learn the mechanisms of the unconscious thought and be able to tell why our engines which we thought we had only to *drive* do not develop as much power as they ought, do not steer as straight or run as smoothly and quietly as they should; and with such a knowledge of the workings of the boy or girl motor car we shall be able to remove the hood, adjust the valve stems, clean the oiler, decarbonize the cylinders, etc., and take as keen a pleasure in being skilful mechanics as we thought to take as chauffeurs. Behind the " shining morning face " there is a much more complicated mechanism than that inside of the polished exterior of the sleek young car direct from the factory. We had somehow got the idea that, as an automobile runs better after about a thousand miles, all we had to do was to " joy-ride " each one a thousand or so and turn it over to the owner a little the better for wear.

Possibly I might better have compared the teacher to an assembler of the parts of the machine. Any child of twelve can run one, if it works properly. But the fact is that the automobile-children that come to our classroom-garage have themselves been run by children mostly before we get them. They have been run without oil till they knock, without everything except gas, and sometimes that was full of water, due to the " fooling " of the people who had the use of the machine before the teacher saw it.

One of the parts of the unconscious thought mechanism treats reality as I have treated the unwilling spirit, weak flesh proposition. It turns reality inside out and hind side before, and, with one of the combinations, sometimes least suited to the conscious purposes of society, it produces a result quite the opposite of that which best adapts the individual to his social environment. Other parts of the unconscious thought mechanism work in other ways and produce other contradictory results. So that what the child does or does not do, says or does not say, in school has to be interpreted as modern psychoanalysis interprets a dream. The dream has a manifest content (its apparent, bizarre narrative), and also a latent content, which never by any chance is visible, except in the youngest children, but which has to be deduced from the manifest content through the thoughts associated with the elements of the manifest content. If my manipulation of the unwilling spirit, etc., seemed futile or uninteresting to some persons, it was because they did not see its intimate connection with the realities which confront us in the schoolroom (as everywhere else). I conversed this morning with a young teacher who confessed to me that she did not teach, she only went through the motions of teaching. I talked the other evening with an old teacher who admitted that teaching had become to him a deadly grind, as indeed why should not driving be to a mere chauffeur? Both of these teachers failed to get the interest out of their profession they would have had if they had seen that teaching is both a science and an art, a science whose sphere is the entirety of human thought, conscious *and* unconscious, and an art whose medium can now, thanks to the newer psychology, be the infinite depths of the human soul. It is my belief that the study of the latent unconscious, as manifested in conscious thought and act, will give to teaching a fascination which artists find in real life and bring into their studios, which novelists find in Vanity Fair, which producers of all kinds find in the problems of their factories and of the means of distributing their products, and which inventors find in their laboratories. By the recognition, and only by the recognition, of the limitless possibilities opened up by the knowledge of some part of the unconscious shall we be able to see the " willing spirit " in the " strong flesh."

Summary

The question as to what act is most personal is answered by calling what we most desire the most intimately our own act. The majority of desires are unconscious ones. Illustrations are given of the unconscious perception by one person of certain personal qualities of another and their evaluation according to primeval standards. A specific instance is cited of the absolutely unconscious factor in a stream of most intense consciousness (adding a column of figures) and attention is called to the fact that even the number three, when it is an idea and not a mere word, is a centre of force. This indicates the possibility of all ideas being dynamic. The simultaneous satisfaction of conscious and unconscious wishes in different spheres of life, including the schoolroom. The unconscious wish enters as an ingredient into every mental activity. Unconscious inference, of the immediate type, is discussed, and the relation between a statement and the unconscious wish brought out. This leads to the view that the contradictory of a proposition is as valuable to the unconscious as the proposition itself, because the negative has no psychological but only a logical value. This is illustrated by the statement that the spirit is willing and the flesh is strong.

CHAPTER III

IT is my present desire to illustrate as many combinations as possible of the conscious and the unconscious act and thought, as they are manifested in the everyday life of child and adult alike. I have omitted from this book any mention of the foreconscious, deeming it unnecessary for the theses of the book, but for the sake of completeness I will add here a brief exposition of its main features. In omitting mention of the foreconscious I have been obliged to increase the connotation of the term unconscious. The unconscious is the repository of all the ideas, sensations, etc., which have ever entered our minds, and possibly of others which have not entered our minds during our own lives, but have been inherited. Of the inheritance of unconscious ideas, however, there is no scientific proof.

The distinction between the unconscious and the foreconscious is that the former contains all the memories, which *cannot* come to consciousness, and there are a great many of them, while the foreconscious contains the memories of all kinds which can be voluntarily evoked from time to time. Between this freely coming and going group of ideas which, like familiar names, dates, telephone numbers, scraps of poetry, music, etc., and the vast body of totally unconscious memories, accumulated certainly during the lifetime of the individual and possibly during the life of the race, there is a barrier over which the truly unconscious mental activities are absolutely unable to pass. We know of their existence by inference only, but by an inference which is so logical and free from fallacy that it is impossible for those to doubt it who have taken the trouble to sift the evidence. Not only of the existence of this unconscious, the thoughts of our minds, irrecoverable, without the special technique of psychoanalysis, but of its nature we have some reliable information. It exists as a blind wish, an amorphous craving which can best be described as an unreasoning urge to life and love. The illimitable power of this desire, expressing itself among other words in minute muscular contractions in all parts of the body, is normally able to transcend the barrier above mentioned only in the form of actions which are approved by society. Certain disguises are adopted by the utterly unconscious *wish,* which convert it into specific foreconscious *wishes* with a definite form, and, bearing these disguises, it comes now and then into full consciousness. The group of disguises, much like the costumes of the actors in a play, and like the words, intonations and movements which are prescribed by the author and the stage manager, are ready in the wings of the foreconscious to appear in the drama of consciousness. And as the author will not write, or the stage manager produce, what will not appeal to the public, so the guardian called the " Censor " at the barrier above mentioned will not allow any unconscious wish to appear, except those disguised so as to be acceptable to society.

Thus is to be represented the condition of thoughts which exist in the permanently unconscious and in the temporarily unconscious state called the foreconscious. But as the concept of the foreconscious is not really necessary to the mere presentation of the unconscious factor in education, I am obliged to omit what, if carried out fully, would occupy a book in itself.

It would be interesting to speculate upon the degree to which even the most conscious ideas which we possess are backgrounded by the wishes of which we are never conscious and to study out the possible relations between the nature of the unconscious element of any wish and its conscious factor.   A thorough investigation of these matters would, I am sure, bring to light a great deal of fact which would explain almost everything in human psychology which is now very difficult to elucidate.

I have already mentioned the fact of the unconscious element which is found interspersed throughout the stream of consciousness, even where it seems to be flowing most narrowly and most swiftly.   Certain relations of the conscious and the unconscious activities, as shown in thought and action, here invite consideration.   And first I regard as unconscious acts both those of which we never become aware, such as the movements of muscles and fluids accompanying the physiological functions which never enter consciousness as such, and the movements of the parts of the body of which we only sometimes become conscious.   Some of these are called symptomatic acts from their analogy with the symptoms of certain nervous diseases, although, as they occur in all persons, well or ill, there is no present implication of abnormality in them.   They are all blunders, errors, slips of the tongue or pen, mannerisms, and even some forms of so-called neuralgia, twitching of the face, etc.

As we are concerned here with four factors, conscious thought, unconscious thought, conscious action and unconscious action and the causal relation existing between them, it will not be a complete consideration of our topic if we leave unmentioned any one of the combinations.

Conscious Action

By conscious action I mean, of course, action of which we are conscious, which includes voluntary action and involuntary movements of which we get a sensational report through the afferent nerves.   The causes of voluntary action may be supposed to be the thoughts which precede and accompany it.   The causes of the involuntary movements have hitherto been presumed to be movements and not thoughts, that is, movements in the tissues of the body.   But it seems quite certain that when movements become small enough they are indistinguishable conceptually from thoughts, which we must therefore include as among the causes of the involuntary muscular movements, as well as of the movements involved in the various physiological functions.   So that we can see here the possibility of the involuntary movements being caused by unconscious thoughts, and we get an idea of how logically necessary is the concept of an unconscious thought, and what may be supposed to be the nature of an unconscious thought—namely, a movement which is so slight that it has not the force to penetrate into consciousness, or, figuratively speaking, the position whence it could pass over into or be read off as conscious thought.   And we see, finally, that the only difference between a conscious thought and an unconscious thought is just this fact of its being in consciousness, its being cognized, our being aware of it. There is no other difference whatever. And we can see that, if we suppose conscious thoughts to be causes of movements, both conscious movements and unconscious movements, there is no reason why we should deny to a thought some causative power, just because it has not happened to enter consciousness. And the fact that it has not entered consciousness does not imply that it is not strong enough to do so, for the newer psychology has shown that the thoughts of which we never are conscious have been opposed in their attempts to enter consciousness by a special barrier set up by the censor, a barrier of special strength, peculiarly adapted to exclude that very thought. And we must suppose that the thought which struggles toward consciousness is progressively strengthened and that the barrier itself is continually piled higher and higher by the censor, so that that particular thought becomes the centre of a battle which is waged by the unconscious against consciousness. Incidentally it may be remarked that such a conflict tends to result eventually in a serious derangement of the physiological functions themselves, leading to both physical and mental disease.

Unconscious Action

By unconscious action I mean, of course, any one of the innumerable motions of and in the body, of which we are generally unconscious, including those of which we sometimes do become aware, the typical instance of which, within the body, is the circulation of the blood. From time to time we do become conscious of the heart-beat and we know how certain kinds of thoughts will cause it to become more rapid. It is also conceivable how certain kinds of thoughts would cause the calibre of the blood vessels to change in different parts of the body, thus lessening or increasing the amount of blood delivered there, and how in the same way other fluids closely connected with the most fundamental physiological processes might be affected.

The greatest possible number of relations existing between the four factors mentioned above is sixteen, as given in the following table:

1. Conscious action causing conscious action,*
2. Conscious action causing conscious thought,
3. Conscious action causing unconscious action,
4. Conscious action causing unconscious thought,
5. Conscious thought causing conscious action,
6. Conscious thought causing conscious thought,*
7. Conscious thought causing unconscious action,
8. Conscious thought causing unconscious thought,
9. Unconscious action causing conscious action,
10. Unconscious action causing conscious thought,
11. Unconscious action causing unconscious action,*
12. Unconscious action causing unconscious thought,
13. Unconscious thought causing conscious action,
14. Unconscious thought causing conscious thought,
15. Unconscious thought causing unconscious action,
16. Unconscious thought causing unconscious thought.*

Nos. 1, 6, 11 and 16, starred in the above list, imply that an action can cause an action and a thought can cause a thought, whether either of them is conscious or uncon-

scious. The question as to the validity of a thought causing a thought is more metaphysical than psychological or
educational, and must in this book be accepted as the basis
from which it is written; also the validity of the statement
that an unconscious thought really exists, as no attempt
will be made in this book to prove it. As for a movement
(action) causing a movement, that is a matter of everyday physics.

The Unconscious and the Conscious Interplay

But the interplay between conscious and unconscious
action and conscious and unconscious thought is a matter
that daily affects the work and conduct in every schoolroom, as it does indeed in every meeting place of humans,
and some phases of this interplay are so important, particularly for teacher and parent, and withal so little
understood, that it is thought advisable here to study
some of them in detail.

In the slip of the tongue we have an example of an
action which at the time of its occurrence was unconscious,
that is, unnoticed by the person making it. Sometimes the
mistake is noticed later and rectified by the person himself,
sometimes it is noticed and corrected by others, and in
this case it is not infrequent that the person making the
slip of the tongue denies that he has made it. The action
may therefore be performed while the person is unaware
of it, and may or may not later be recognized by the same
person. It is different with slips of the pen, which are of
course automatically registered. The mistake is in this
case recorded and there can be no question as to its having actually been made.

In both cases what was unconscious comes later into consciousness. But in both cases the action has been unconscious, and in no sense can we say that it was caused by conscious thought or action. It must therefore be the effect of an unconscious factor. Whether that cause be an action or a thought is not of any great importance, the only significant aspect of it being that it had a cause in the unconscious part of the mind.

While from one point of view it makes no difference whether the unconscious factor is a thought or an action, for the purpose of schematic completeness I will include mention of unconscious actions which produce or cause conscious thoughts. Unconscious actions producing unconscious actions and thoughts are conceivable as absolutely continuous in all life from the beginning to the end of it. For by unconscious actions we mean all the physiological processes, and many of the larger motions of the parts of the body.

Clues to the mental effects of physiological (i.e. unconscious) causes are given us in the mental effects of certain drugs, e.g. quinine producing an auditory sensation and hasheesh producing a visual sensation, and so on through the emetics, sudorifics, etc., named according to the ways in which their effects enter consciousness.

As to the mental (here meaning conscious) effects of unconscious mental activities, the newer psychology here furnishes us with facts many of which appear at first paradoxical, and all of them are highly important for the teacher and the parent. For it seems quite reasonable, when our attention is called to it, to say that, if there are so many and so constant influences of the physiological processes upon the conscious, and even more upon the unconscious thoughts, there is more than a mere likelihood that unconscious thoughts themselves have an influence over conscious ones. It is inconceivable indeed that all the sights, sounds and other impressions we have had, and all the thoughts, ideas and feelings we have ever experienced, which are stored in the unconscious portion of the mind, should *not* have an effect upon each other and so upon our present nervous constitution, and thereby determine the nature, if not the existence, of the thoughts which come to us from time to time.

Clearly, then, the unconscious thoughts, thoughts we have had consciously and then allowed to slip, or forcibly expelled, from consciousness, are ever present in the great and always developing world of the unconscious, and, by their unnoticed activities, they colour our every present conscious thought. And so we can go on and, once having had our attention called to it, detect the unconscious factor in all human action, a bit of detective work which is exceedingly fascinating, but which has to be carried on with the greatest caution and the results rarely, if ever, communicated, because they are, for a very good reason, strenuously rejected, and particularly by the persons in whom they are detected. A little practice in this picking out of the unconscious factor in the acts and thoughts of ourselves and our fellows soon shows us, too, how extremely great is the ratio which it bears to the conscious factor.

Conscious Control of Unconscious Thoughts

On the other side, however, is the possibility of the conscious thoughts causing unconscious ones, of the conscious life influencing the unconscious life within us.* This is indeed one of, if not the most important of, the aims of education in general. Without the assumption that conscious activity has an effect on us, there would be no use in an attempt to educate. But what can be the effect, if it is not an effect on the unconscious thoughts and, through them, on the unconscious actions? And here lies also another implication, namely that, if there is a causal connection between unconscious thoughts and unconscious actions, which include the physiological processes, why may the connection not work both ways? Why may it not be possible that a well-learned lesson may be as conducive to good digestion, for instance, as a violent toothache impedes the learning of it?

It seems in every way more rational to suppose that conscious and unconscious thought and action are causally connected in both directions, in addition to the consideration that training of every kind is but the conscious control of unconscious activity, whether movement or thought.

Unconscious Control of Unconscious

We come finally to the question of the causal relation between the unconscious factors themselves. In this connection it is plain that the thoughts outside of consciousness influence each other without let or hindrance. They grow as in an untended garden, or one tended (up to the present age) by merely the fractional attention that a

---

*Dewey (*Democracy and Education,* page 188) says that no idea can be transmitted from one mind to another, and (page 272) that much of experience is indirect. If that be true, it is all the more advisable for all those interested in the welfare of humanity to learn the means, most penetrating into human nature, of helping society in its development along the line of conquering chaos with consciousness.

very narrowly limited ability to bring them into consciousness can exercise. What goes on below the threshold of consciousness in each and every soul is, at first glance, appalling to contemplate. There is no doubt, too, that the appalling nature of it has been the deterrent factor operating to turn men's gaze away from it for so many centuries. But as with all deterrent things, the fear it inspires vanishes on closer inspection. There is also no question that to any person, when he first entertains the thought of the unkemptness of his own (and everyone's else) unconscious, there seems to be nothing in the world so shameful, so savage, so hopeless. But that feeling soon passes, giving way to one which makes clear one of the central aims of education, namely, to make possible the widest scope of conscious life, to enable each individual to realize as fully as possible what he actually is, inside and out, so to speak, and incidentally what other persons are. We become then better acquainted, as it were, all around, and more likely to make allowances for each other.

And as a fundamental purpose of academic education I believe this one stands out pre-eminent, namely, to enable each individual to take at will into consciousness as many and as diverse thoughts as possible which the uneducated person is unable to face. For this aim, expressed in other words, is to enable the individual to face as much reality as possible. And in this I may at first seem to be implying that the unconscious is the same as reality, or that the only reality is the unconscious. But it is easy to see how that might be true, or how it becomes true, if the individual develops naturally and without help from the outside.

For the innate tendency of all individuals, from the earliest days of infancy, is to repress reality, to forget it voluntarily, to drive it from consciousness and keep it out of consciousness, because reality is largely, and more and more in nervous persons than in others, a source of pain and distress. The first painful experience of the infant is annihilated for it by a wriggle, or disposed of by crying until some other hand removes the painful thing, and this attitude of rejection is typical of all repression. But there is no question any longer about the fate of such repressed experiences. They are not really annihilated, as the infant might think, but are driven back into its own unconscious. And so we go on from year to year, accumulating in the unconscious all the painful and distressing experiences. By doing so we make them non-existent only as far as consciousness is concerned.

Repressing the Neurotic

Neurotics are those persons for whom the world of external reality is only or largely a source of distress. This being the case the neurotic is the trouble finder who is at any rate the forerunner, if not the actual elaborator of improvements. All progress is improvement. All improvement in social relations implies the need of improvement. The assertion of that need is loudly disclaimed by society, because of the natural inertia of humanity. The specialization of the neurotic is needed to furnish the push that is necessary to steer society from the direction in which, with gyroscopic fidelity, it is heading, and cause those deviations without which society would remain a permanent crystallization. Society, without

the nervous activity of the neurotic which it at first represses and later digests, would never develop beyond
the most rudimentary form.

The import of all this for teachers is plain. If the
children, or some of them, who are before the teacher,
belong to the neurotic type, as undoubtedly some do in
every school, they will be children whom the teacher
cannot handle in the way in which he has to handle the
others. The same external uniformity, so far as democratic institutions may demand, will have to be maintained,
but the mental attitude of the teacher will necessarily be
somewhat different in the case of the two groups. In view
of the fact that the neurotic children are destined to
furnish the variations from the regular so-called norm of
humanity and become as it were the models of the society
of the future, the teacher will have to devote a somewhat
more special interest to this group. In the neurotic boy
or girl there will be the possibility of developing the
ideas which society will later adopt. Any capriciousness
of such children will have to be given a certain amount of
respect. The strange ideas which such children may
express are not to be ridiculed by the teacher, who in
ridiculing them would be in the position of the barking
dog which uses this method of heralding everything
strange. It is the proper province of the dog, but not that
of the thoughtful human.

There is, however, a perfectly rational explanation of
every whimsy of every child. It is the duty of the teacher
to examine into the causes of everything in the nature of
the erratic in children's behaviour and see where the
logic of the situation lies. Much injustice is done to
children if their thoughts are not given the attention they

deserve.   By ridiculing the unusual expressions of children, or by thoughtlessly brushing them aside as irrelevant, teachers do much wrong both to the children and to themselves, because the amount of attention given to the really original thoughts of the children is more than paid for by the new point of view which the teacher may thereby gain.   If the teacher in ignoring the peculiarities of the children, adheres rigidly to the inelastic requirements of the curriculum, he will be required himself to devote all the time of himself and his class to the slavish following out of the prescribed details.   If he never made any variation in treatment, of course he could never make any progress.   If the curriculum is framed with the greatest care to fill the needs of the majority of the pupils, it will not suit at least a small minority.   This minority is by all odds the most interesting, and in the end the most progressive, because it is from them that the variations are to come which will form the still developing norm of future generations.

There will be the added satisfaction for the teacher, if he has some regard for the peculiarities of the minority of children, that he may be the means of reducing their maladaptation to their environment.   For instance, the peculiar child is always attacked either literally or figuratively by the other children in the class, who laugh at him, or even fly at him physically.   If the teacher, holding as he may legitimately the point of view that the irregular child is not going to get on so smoothly in the world, and that his irregularities will be at least a slight burden to him, attempts to prune away and suppress all the peculiarities of the child in the effort to make him perfectly *normal,* he is of course doing exactly what the children themselves are unconsciously trying to do, and he thereby reduces himself to their level, which is that of the fixed social environment. Now, the function of the neurotic in society, being to change, through his own variability, the uniformity of the social fabric as a whole, should be favoured by the teacher and not obstructed. Obstructing the changes suggested by the actions and thought of the unusual child will be doing the teacher's best to go against the development of society. As the aim of education is the adaptation of the individual to the social environment, this includes also the possibility that the environment may be a changing one and not fixed. If that is the case, the very worst thing that the teacher could do is to add a crystallizing force to the flux of social life, for in so doing he is himself obstructing and not helping the progress of social development.

The actions of the peculiar or unusual child are in a sense quite analogous to the thoughts emanating from the unconscious which the conscious life is constantly attempting to repress. In fact, the thoughts and actions of the neurotic in general are much more likely to be a more direct expression of the unconscious than are those of the so-called normal. If it is the duty of the individual to recognize and adapt himself to the greatest amount of unconscious life, it is surely that of the teacher not to ignore but to study the manifestations of the unconscious as they are developed in the children above and below the average of intelligence, as it is called. If the teacher simply ignores the actions of the neurotic child, or, failing to be able to ignore them, succeeds in repressing them, he is doing for humanity at large exactly what every individual is doing for himself, and sometimes to his great disadvantage, for he is rejecting at least one form of reality.

The tendency on the part of the individual to repress the unpleasant or the difficult or even the unusual elements in his life is irresistible in childhood, relieved only sporadically by masochism.*

It is as if the unconscious of the child were a magnet which attracted pleasure and repelled pain. And it is as if the pleasure were attracted to one part of its soul, while the repelled pain drifted not away from the personality entirely but toward another part of it, the unconscious. It must be so, for we cannot conceive otherwise than that the human organism is a perfect and complete register of *all* the external world with which it comes in contact, and that if some of the experiences are locked up, finally, in a portion of the organism so securely that they cannot be accessible to consciousness, they are nevertheless *in the mind,* and their effects are, though different, as real as they would be if the individual could succeed in reaching them. They are indeed the reflection, the personal complement, of a good portion of reality, and the individual who cannot, or dare not, look at them or take them into consciousness and become aware of them at will is, so to speak, only a fractional personality. But most of us are that. This is what I mean therefore by saying that the unconscious is the reality within us. It is the other side of experience, absorbed into the mind, and by most persons sedulously ignored because of its unpleasantness.

The aim of education therefore being to develop the fullest personality, we inevitably conclude that the means

* See page 89.

to this end is the re-cognizing (cognizing again) what has been repressed into the unconscious.   It has been cognized once, when it was received into consciousness the first time, but the tendency to repress unpleasant experiences is always so strong that we finally succeed in keeping them out of consciousness (though not out of mind) forever.

So complete is the repression of the undesired elements of experience that for most people it is absolutely impossible, unaided, ever to recover these elements, although it has been found, in medical psychoanalysis, that the recovery of the memories of unpleasant experiences has frequently been the means of a recovery from mental or physical ills.   Therefore the word recovery takes on a new significance, meaning, as it does, the regaining both of banished thoughts and of the entirety of reality, and, at the same time, the recovery of health (Health=wholth). Perfect health means the ability to do anything that is humanly possible up to the maximum efficiency of the individual organism.   It means also the ability to accept any idea, whatever its source.   When for any reason the individual thinks he is unable to eat and do anything, or is unable to entertain certain kinds of ideas, his personal entirety is beginning to acquire limitations.   He begins to lose his wholeness, that is, his health.   And there is no question that this attitude is at least quite as much mental as physical.   What tells a dyspeptic that he cannot digest this or that?   Certainly not his body directly. He makes mental inferences about reports from his body, and they are usually erroneous inferences.

The Combinations

To resume, after this lengthy digression, the consideration of the relations of the four factors mentioned on page 54, we find that

1.*

2. Conscious action causing conscious thought is illustrated by ordinary perception. The sensation of blue and violet colours on the distant horizon and green and yellow nearby is automatically interpreted as, for instance, a road between trees with a mountain against the blue sky in the background. I take it that the conscious action of sensation causes the conscious thought " mountain." It is quite evident, however, that the immediate effect is more than fully described in these words. For if we carry on the train of thought suggested by " mountain " we have thought upon thought occurring to the mind, all supplied by the unconscious and mediated by its fundamental creative wish, all of which mental phenomena are not the direct effects of the mountain view alone.

3. Conscious action causing unconscious action is illustrated by the things we do all the time, things of which we are not aware, when these can be traced to the actions we are then doing. Possibly the best illustration is the physiological changes accomplished by the body in its preparation for an emergency which is reported to consciousness at the same time. For instance, the actions of the limbs in the event of stumbling, or better yet the changes in circulation, respiration, etc., occurring when one is really or ideally preparing for a physical struggle, and we

* Discussed above, page 54.

know from recent researches that these are very elaborate and far-reaching.

Unconscious action caused by conscious action is amply illustrated by the mannerisms of all people. When they talk or work they do certain things with their hands, for instance, of which they are generally quite unconscious. Much of the study of motions in manufacturing operations has been devoted to the eliminating of these wasted motions, which might have been removed quite as effectively, if not as speedily, by means of a mental analysis of the operatives, as all these useless motions are the expression of the unconscious wish not to be efficient. If this wish had been understood and removed, the useless motions would have vanished without further effort. This and No. 9 are probably not pure cases, because all actions are generally, if not always, mediated through ideas, either conscious ones or unconscious ones.

4. Conscious action causing unconscious thought is what we try to effect in academic education. Not only is it an aim of education to increase the amount of unconscious material which consciousness can take in and assimilate, but it is a further aim of education to exercise some control over the organism (or organic unity) constituting the unconscious. The advantage of this control is obvious if it can be attained, for otherwise the control is that of the conscious life by the unconscious, the latter in most people completely dominating the former. If such control over the unconscious by the conscious cannot be gained, education loses its main advantage. For the assumption that education has the function of passing on to the individual the experience, in condensed form, of the race is based upon the other assumption that the expe-

rience of the race can find some lodgment in the mind of the individual. And this lodgment can be effected only through the assimilation of the experience of the race *by* the individual unconscious. It comes by various paths, but all through conscious ones and mostly verbal. But if the *unconscious* of the individual is, through early environment, *made inaccessible to* conscious influences, then the task of educating that individual becomes infinitely more onerous than it would otherwise have been, perhaps even impossible. And it is one of the theses of this book that, because of the ignorance of parents, for which they are in no sense to blame, *the unconscious of a large number of school children has been made inaccessible to conscious influences,* so that almost all the work of the teacher is absolutely fruitless.

In short, we may say that unconscious thoughts caused by conscious action is the name of a continuous stream of influence which works upon the unconscious daily. It is the only way by which we can control the enormous power of the unconscious desire. Comparatively little knowledge that is definite and ready for application to our present system of education is available as yet, but the small portion which is, should be spread and used as if it were a particle of radium, for it is able to accomplish what no other agency in the world can, except the conscious thought which is directed intelligently to gain control of and to socialize the great power of the unconscious.

5. Conscious thought causing conscious action is what we all know as voluntary action. We desire and will and act, and the first of these causes the second and the second the third. There is nothing new in this.

6.*

7. Conscious thought causing unconscious action is common in the generally recognized influence of mind over body. That unconscious thought causes unconscious action, however, is not included in the general proposition that mind influences body.

Unconscious action caused by conscious thought is seen in the symptomatic action following certain perceptions. The fidgeting about when an emergency occurs, the clearing of one's throat when, in preparing to make a speech, one thinks of the possibility of making a mistake, and much coughing in congregations and school assemblies are an expression of unconscious thoughts of disapproval of some element of the " exercises."

Consciousness is evidently much more limited in its scope than action. There are, in other words, actions which are so rapid and so numerous that for consciousness they exist only as groups. Thus unconscious action caused by conscious thought is seen in everything we *learn to do*. Playing a piece on a piano is a concrete example of conscious thought producing actions so rapid that there can be no consciousness of them as separate entities. Speaking a foreign language is another. The conscious thought sets in motion parts of our bodies (lips, throat, etc.) of which we are not specifically aware. The attempt to become conscious of a single element while it is taking place in one of these groups of which we are conscious only as of a group, sometimes results in a failure of the group to be carried out successfully. Thus, if we are running downstairs, it is frequently disastrous to attend separately to the motions necessary to take one

* Discussed, p. 54.

of the steps, because the consciousness which should be given to the whole flight is suddenly taken away from the whole flight as a unit.

Mistakes in playing the piano come from this irregular shift of the attention, which is equivalent to saying from a shift of consciousness from a larger to a smaller unit. This shows very clearly why it is disadvantageous to attempt to play a piece of music at a rapid tempo until all the motions of the fingers and hands have become so firmly associated that the individual motions can be left safely to the unconscious. We thus also see the true advantage of constant practice, and just what practice does. It hands over the control of the motions from consciousness to the unconscious (that part of it which is called the foreconscious). The thoughts which were in consciousness, and necessarily there during the learning of the piece, or of the groups of motions of which it is composed, are dropped back into the unconscious and become unconscious thoughts, and it is these unconscious thoughts which function in producing the mechanical operations, while consciousness itself is devoted to the relations of tempo, intensity, tone quality, etc., which are determined in turn by other unconscious thoughts connected with still wider aspects of the ego, i.e. various desires for superiority, etc., which are struggling for gratification during the performance of the piece.

Quite the same process goes on in literary composition, where the conscious motions of writing with the pen, or on the typewriter, are caused partly by the conscious thoughts which the writer is trying to express, and partly by the unconscious thoughts which are continually struggling for outward expression. This combination of effort between consciousness and the unconscious in literary composition always results in a compromise, what is actually written being a result of both causes combined. The actual effect of the unconscious cause in this case is primarily the selection of the words used. It is quite evident that the actual words occur, apparently of their own accord, although a selection of several possibilities may well seem to be the work of consciousness itself. This is illustrated by the fact that a poet is frequently unable to give any reason for the use of a given word in his poem, when asked to do so. " It just came; it was the only word that fitted," etc., may be the non-committal reply.

In those who use pen or machine with absolute fluency, writing is an example of a group of motions whose separate elements are as far as possible removed from consciousness, which is devoted to quite other aims, frequently indeed following a definite affect or emotion, and allowing first the words to come into consciousness, sifted through the conscious purpose, and yet not in the least determining the words or the grammatical forms which are offered by the unconscious wish. So completely is consciousness segregated from the actual motions that frequently they are imperfectly carried out. A word is misspelled or entirely omitted, two words will coalesce (as " withe " for " with the "), which consciousness perceives neither as a faulty action nor as a defective visual impression.

8. Conscious thought causing unconscious thought is a concept contributed by the newer medical psychology. This, too, is one of the major aims of education, and, although the distinction between unconscious action and unconscious thought is so hard to draw, on account of the approximation of both thought and action to each other in

the unconscious (see page 52), it must be mentioned in this place as well as in the other. Unconscious ideas are caused by, or at any rate modified by, conscious ideas continually in our mental life. In infancy or early childhood we make erroneous inferences about four of the most vital of human relations,—fatherhood, motherhood, sisterhood, brotherhood, and even marriage,—causing unconscious ideas which, in turn, later affect every important decision we make about the matters most intimate to us.

The fact that conscious thought may cause changes in unconscious thought may be objected to by the persons who declare that unconscious thought or unconscious mental activity has no existence. I think it has been amply demonstrated, however, not only that unconscious thought is not a contradiction in terms, and equivalent to unconscious consciousness, but that its nature is that of continuous wish or tension, one of whose aspects is that of a tension, muscular in quality, which nevertheless is potentially a conscious sensation or perception. Accepting this position we are forced to admit that the causal relation may work quite as well one way as the other; in other words, not only that a conscious thought may cause changes in the thoughts or tensions, both those which have never been in consciousness and those which have been but are so no longer, but also that the unconscious tensions or mental activities may have an effect upon the conscious states of mind. This is actually the most important, because the most constant and frequent of the influences which affect conscious life, an influence which has not been known to exist or, even if suspected, had so much of an air of mystery about it that it baffled all previous investigators. But now that the modes of activity (or so-called mechanisms) in which this unconscious desire operates in itself and controls at the same time the operations of conscious thought are beginning to be known, a great deal of the apparent inconsistency and capriciousness of human nature is comprehensible and reducible to known natural laws. Thus the existence of unconscious mental activity and the possibility of creating changes in it, training it to work in desirable modes and to align itself with the purposes of real civilization, gives an entirely new aspect to the problems of education. If we have in us, and are ordinarily dominated by, a group of continuous tensions all striving to manifest themselves to consciousness, or even merely to issue from a state of tension into a condition of actual movement which constitutes their relation, and if the tendency to issue into actual movement takes the form of an action not congruent with the social environment of the individual, as it does when the instincts urge him to commit selfish acts, then the sooner we can learn how to direct these mere tensions which constitute the unconscious of everyone the better. In order to do this successfully we shall have to revise a great deal of our educational theory as it stands today in order to make it conform with the new facts as we discover them from time to time.

9. Unconscious action causing conscious action is familiar as perception accompanied by automatic movement, which later enters consciousness. Involuntary blinking and all other similar acts are illustrations. Conscious action caused by unconscious action is illustrated by the attempt to suppress or control mannerisms such as stroking the beard. The causing of conscious action by uncon-

scious action is of course the story of all movement in the
physical world.   But for the entrance of consciousness
at some time during the period of evolution there would
be no conscious mentality in the world.   We suppose that
during the course of evolution the element of consciousness entered; but we have no means of knowing how or
when, and we can but speculate on the reason why.   It
has been surmised by some that it entered at the point
where an awkwardness or difficulty arose in the combinations of matter and force, a difficulty such that comparison and preference resulted, and that the need for more
and wider consciousness grew as combinations became
more complicated, difficulties more numerous and the
need for finer adaptations became greater.   At that point
in the course of evolution when consciousness did enter as
a factor in the causal nexus it became *ipso facto* capable
of being a cause itself and an effect of other causes.   So
that wherever it appears, it is itself the effect either of a
physical or a mental cause or the cause of some other
physical or mental state.

The unconscious action which causes the conscious
action most familiar to common observation is ordinary
sensation.   The vibration of the ether, which is unconscious action, causes through the sympathetic nervous
system the adaptations of the eye which give us the sensation of light.   Similarly the quite unconscious chemical
action of quinine gives us the conscious sensation of a
ringing in the ears.   The actual external motion consequent on the perception of the light is, however, the
movements in the muscles of the iris of the eye and
those controlling the convexity of the lens.   The action
of doing something appropriate to the light or the drug,

and not the sensation, is considered by some to be the result of the light or the drug, and the sensation itself to be merely an epiphenomenon. But to such people consciousness of every kind is epiphenomenal and as such is excluded from the causal nexus, but its substratum the disposition is admitted.

10. Unconscious action causing conscious thought we see in anyone's becoming aware of having made a mistake, in his feeling a bodily pain of any kind or in any way becoming aware of any of his own physiological processes. Also it is seen in any conscious reflection about any instinctive acts. This variety of awareness is particularly poignant about the time of puberty, when physical changes that have taken place or are taking place are brought into the consciousness of the adolescent in terms which he or she is unable at first to understand. Here too education's task, which has been most inadequately performed in the past, places a new responsibility in the hands of the teacher, which those not having some knowledge of the unconscious will hardly be able to fulfil.

The instincts and the instinctive acts are *par excellence* the unconscious acts which cause conscious thoughts because of their peculiarly compelling nature. The conscious thoughts experienced as reactions to these instinctive actions, particularly during the period of adolescence, are with some individuals so unfortunate as to mar to some extent their entire subsequent life. The new powers arising from the unifying of the reproductive functions under the primacy of the genital zone * are so great, and the fortuitous and undirected employment of them frequently so disastrous, that it seems as if edu-

* Compare the author's *Man's Unconscious Conflict,* page 128.

cation had no more important task than successfully to pilot the adolescent through this period.

Other examples of conscious thoughts caused by unconscious actions are all such ideas as may occur to anyone, as, for instance, that it would be really better to correct one's habits. Unconscious action may be said to cause conscious thought in all cases where we become conscious of actions after we have performed them. This applies, of course, to the sudden awareness of having made a blunder or blurted out a truth we had intended to conceal, or finally become conscious of the real significance of our actions, many of which we perform first and realize the meaning of only afterwards. This becoming aware of the inner significance of our actions is a sort of waking up, an illumination, a sudden burst of realization that we have builded better than we know (or worse), and indeed is illustrated by all instances where we suddenly become aware of the unconscious factor in our conscious actions. The unconscious element in all conscious action has already been mentioned in another section (9), and I believe the most valuable thoughts that ever come to us are those which make us aware of this unconscious element. This is an awareness that poignantly gives meaning to what was before meaningless. And the results of this kind of awareness are very noticeable in the health and happiness of the individual. Nowhere else is it so clear that ignorance is darkness and that in darkness is disease and disorder of every kind. And no kind of disease is so charged with misery as that which springs from an unenlightened state of the creative craving. Many a person has lived a life darkened by a misinterpretation of, or by a failure to understand, this most vital of all desires, and to see it in its true relations to himself and particularly to herself, and to society.

11.*

12. Unconscious action causing unconscious thought is also a new concept contributed by the later analytical psychology. The existence of this variety of human experience is naturally impossible to sense directly. The results of it fill conscious experience, but the actuality of it is necessarily a matter of inference.

In the sphere of instinct these unconscious actions must inevitably produce unconscious thoughts which are of the greatest moment to the individual life.

13. Unconscious thought causing conscious action we find in a great many situations where the individual is at a loss to explain why he did thus and so. In fact, all such actions can be explained only on the supposition that they were caused by unconscious thought or action. A phobia or any other unreasonable fear is an illustration in ordinary life, and, in the schoolroom, any unwillingness or any irresistible impulse on the part of the child to do any particular thing or not to do it has to be thus accounted for. It can be explained in no other way than that this conscious action was caused by some unconscious thought.

As will be shown in the section on rationalization (page 164), an inability to assign the proper reason for a conscious action is characteristic of persons of all ages, however much they may be willing to give some reason. The reasons assigned by most people for their religion, their political views and their ideas about sex are all really supplied by unconscious thoughts, no matter how strongly

* Discussed page 58.

the persons may affirm that the given reasons are the real ones.

Conscious action caused by unconscious thought is illustrated by a great deal of the thoughtless action so characteristic of humans, adults as well as children, and when occurring in extreme form is known to neurologists as compulsion.

Conscious action is caused by unconscious thought (that is, unconscious wishes, because all unconscious thoughts are wishes or tendencies). In a certain degree all of our conscious acts are partly determined by our unconscious thoughts. Those acts which we consider to be the most completely dominated by consciousness, where indeed we seem to will everything we do, exactly according to a definite conscious plan, are nevertheless not without a large determining factor which comes directly from the unconscious wish. Any mistake or error which we make in doing anything to which we think we are giving our entire attention is absolute proof that that particular act constituting the mistake was not in consciousness at the actual time of the making of the motion. This is true whether the motion be a lip movement, a respiration, a tongue movement, a movement of the hand or a step. It is thus seen that every error, no matter in what sphere of activity it occurs, is an expression of some unconscious wish. This statement seems very paradoxical when the error is a serious blunder leading to illness or loss of life, but it nevertheless remains true in all cases. The unconscious wish which may cause an action leading to loss, as for instance when one fails to lock the stable door and the horse is stolen, may not be, and frequently is not, a definite wish for that kind of result. It may be an un-

conscious wish for something quite different and uncon-
nected with the loss of a horse or anything else. It might
well be an unconscious wish which was for leaving everything wide open, exposed, unprotected, a wish which may
be really a resistance against authority and symbolize the
general desire for superiority. Or an awkward movement which results in knocking a vase from a mantelpiece
and thus breaking a valuable piece of bric-à-brac may or
may not be the expression of a wish to destroy that particular piece. Freud gives, in his *Psychopathology of
Everyday Life,* an excellent example where a statue was
smashed by an awkward movement, where, however, there
was a definite wish in the unconscious to get rid of that
very statue.

Examples of conscious action having nothing but conscious thought as their cause are really impossible to find.
Every conscious action contains so large an element of unconscious thought that it is frequently possible to state
that the conscious element in the causation of it was very
slight indeed. In errors it is, of course, *nil,* and therefore we should perhaps consider this relation under the
head of "unconscious action caused by unconscious
thought." But this rubric I wish to reserve for the perfectly automatic actions which will be discussed under
No. 15.

So that the conscious action caused by unconscious
thought which is seen in errors is really a slight misnomer.
We call the error conscious simply because we become conscious of it as kinetic sensations during or after its performance, in a series of acts to which we are devoting our
"whole attention."

I have been much impressed by the nature of the mistakes made by pupils in the study of a foreign language. The pupil who sees the word " impetum " and reads it " imperium," a word which has occurred a few lines before, is, in this error, possibly expressing an unconscious wish not to exert himself mentally enough to make the fine discrimination necessary to differentiate the words. Those, on the other hand, who never confuse " virīs " with " vīrēs " or " viris " give evidence of an unconscious wish to make such discriminations and are likely to show the same tendency to discriminate finely in other spheres. Of course, the unconscious wishes of all pupils are almost uniformly against making the mental effort to carry on a train of " directed thinking," * instead of floating on the stream of " undirected thinking " or phantasy, where they get without effort the ideal fulfilment of all their unconscious wishes.

The Source of Thoughts

14. Unconscious thought causing conscious thought is illustrated by the foregoing to some extent, but more specifically by the natural occurrence of apparently fanciful ideas during a state of reverie. The occurrence of any idea to the mind from the mind and not from some sensation or perception is a case where a conscious thought is caused or evoked by an unconscious thought.

It is probably not strictly and literally true to say that a conscious thought is caused by *one* unconscious thought, because it is frequently found that the conscious thought is the combined result of several or many unconscious thoughts, each containing a small amount of the gen-

* Cf. page 188.

eral tendency or trend of the unconscious as a whole. It is, however, a fact that every conscious thought which cannot be directly traced to a conscious action, and the only ones that can are the sensations and perceptions, has its real origin in the unconscious. The universality of this rule makes it of the greatest import for education because conscious thoughts which are expressed in conscious acts are the most palpable proof of the results of education, and it is clear that, in order to exercise the best kind of control upon the thoughts which spontaneously occur to the individual, we must devise some means of controlling the source from which the ideas (and ultimately the acts) come in each individual case.

But until teachers and parents realize the uniform source of all ideas (namely, the unconscious), it will be impossible to plan any method which shall exercise the proper control over the source of ideas.

The fact that unconscious thought or tension has an effect upon conscious thought has been suspected for many centuries, but its mechanisms, as recently observed by analytical psychologists in America and Europe, are just today beginning to be understood so that a procedure can be followed out by means of them which will result in a better ability to control them. In short, the unconscious, long unknown, like an undiscovered mine in each and every one of us, is believed to be rich in most valuable ore, which can be worked with profit as soon as the veins are adequately surveyed, and the methods of the reduction of the ore are fully devised.

But more like " a woman in the case " the unconscious mental activity causes actions which are explainable on no other basis than that there is an unconscious mental activity of very high potentiality, and that it furnishes the springs of action which have hitherto baffled the speculation of the most penetrating philosophers.

The most striking contribution of the newer psychology to the knowledge of human conduct was made by its discovery that the ordinary night dream is a direct effect of the unconscious wish, and that instead of being a trivial and insignificant occurrence, it is the straightest road directly into the heart of the unconscious. A dream is *par excellence* the conscious thought caused by the unconscious thought. It is the conscious thought to which no other cause save the unconscious can be attributed. In it we see the unconscious working with the fewest obstructions it finds anywhere in mental life. The only inhibition exercised upon it is by the censor, to pass which all the transformations take place that are effected in the unconscious wish in order to make it presentable as a conscious one.

15. Unconscious thought causing unconscious action is seen in the disorders having a nervous origin which the newer medical psychology has taken as its peculiarly appropriate task to cure. This relation is of only admonitory import to teachers, for it will seldom, if ever, be their duty to attempt to cure the nervousness of a child by the radical method used in psychoanalysis. But all teachers should know that the unconscious thoughts of children and adults are admitted, by a rapidly increasing school of physicians, to be the causes of both mental and physical diseases, many of which have previously been attributed to merely physical causes. The theory of these physicians is that, when the actual unconscious thought, or group of thoughts (called a complex), is accurately

ascertained, the cause of the disease is removed by being brought from the unconscious into consciousness. But it is an impossible task for the average teacher, as indeed it is for some physicians, to find this complex, because it has to be deduced from the voluntary confessions (free associations) of the patient, and *it is never discovered by questioning*. There is hardly a possible question that does not contain a suggested answer, except the one query: " What do you think? " and the answer is most likely to be: " Nothing." I include this relation only for the sake of completeness of inventory, so to speak, the full discussion of it requiring a special treatise.

Unconscious actions are generally caused by unconscious thoughts. The unconscious action of stroking the beard or the chin, pulling the moustache, sticking fingers in buttonholes, rolling up paper, pamphlets, etc., into tight rolls, picking nose, scratching the head, have all been traced to their unconscious causes in the desire for creation, the desire for creation in reproductive forms * being repressed and that for creation in productive form not having been developed in such people to such a degree as to absorb that portion of the primal urge which is leaking out into these so-called symptomatic actions.

That an unconscious thought should be the cause of an unconscious act does not seem strange when once we have admitted the principle of causation into psychology and admitted the existence of the unconscious thought. As we know that the unconscious thought is a tension which is always struggling for expression in action, it is not surprising if some of the numerous tensions of which we are not, and never can become, conscious, gain their

* See page 196.

outlet into external reality through motions, attitudes, mannerisms, facial expressions and grimaces of which also we are generally totally unconscious. On this principle we know that the nervous coughing and clearing of the throat, together with all forms of embarrassment, including stammering and blunders of speech and action, are but the outward manifestation (a very much transformed one) of the primal urge for creation, an issue (not to say a leak) of energy which, in other environment, might have been used up in reproductive or productive creation.

It is noteworthy that from this point of view many of the great accomplishments of humans are examples of unconscious activities, because they are results of which the producer never even dreamed. They are quite analogous, in their formation, to the nervous mannerisms of lesser people. The ideal expenditure of the energy of a man or a woman would consist in that form and degree of productive and reproductive creation which best developed the innate powers of the individuals and prolonged the life of themselves and their families and contributed most to the liberation of the energies of their fellow-men and women, most of which are now being checked by the awkward relations which society, as it has evolved, has imposed upon itself.

In an absolutely healthy development of social relations the numerous inhibitions by which a life in a highly complex form of society is surrounded, makes it very difficult to keep a wholesome balance between the accepted and the unaccepted varieties of relaxation of tensions. Expressed in other words, the unconscious wish for creation meets obstructions on every side, and the more complicated the social environment of the individual the more

numerous are the inhibitions.   Naturally and instinctively
the child seeks to create, and at the time of puberty there
is an almost irresistible urge to reproductive creation.
Education, dimly sensing the need for a transmutation of
this reproductive urge, has, though with comparatively
small success, attempted to employ the creative energies
of men in a productive rather than in a merely reproductive way.   In this, education has to go against instinct, and in this conflict arise the main difficulties of
educational practice.

Unconscious thoughts (which are all wishes) are the
causes of all the unconscious acts which make up so
large a proportion of human conduct, the more youth-
ful the individual the more unconscious the act.   For
a fully conscious act must have in it some element of an
idea of its result.   Take, for example, the throwing of
a stone.   It is of course impossible to say that the boy
who throws a stone is unconscious of what he is doing,
for while he is surely conscious of what he *wants* to do
in throwing the stone, he is unaware of all he is actually
doing, that is, he does not know whether he is going
to hit the right or the wrong thing with it.   He sometimes resolutely blinds himself to the possibility of the
stone's going astray and hitting something with destructive effect.

Careful consideration shows us that there is an unconscious element in every act, as we frequently do or
say things with, for instance, a conscious purpose of
pleasing, when a choice of words, on the spur of the
moment, a choice of words which we are pleased to call
unlucky, spoils the whole effect.   Du Maurier in the
London *Punch* illustrated a series of jokes which ran

for years under the title of " Things Which One Would Rather Have Expressed Differently." The utter failure of such remarks, from the conscious point of view, consists in the unconscious element of the action, an unconscious element which is contributed by the unconscious thought or tension. This unconscious wish may be so hostile to the conscious desire of making a complimentary speech that it completely changes the remark, which was intended to be ingratiating, into a statement most uncomplimentary. In this case we clearly see the unconscious element in the conscious act and the fact that it was caused by the unconscious thought, i.e. wish. Unconscious thoughts, then, do cause actions which are entirely unconscious, as are the mannerisms, and also actions which contain an unconscious element, as do all blunders or actions erroneously carried out. Find and study the unconscious element in your conscious actions, and you take a step toward the understanding of your own unconscious.

It may be said that a great, indeed by far the greatest, part of our several actions and behaviours and our aggregate conduct is composed of this unconscious element. Education in the future will, I think, enable teachers to disentangle these unconscious elements from the actions of their pupils, and thus be able to handle them better. In the still more distant future, direct instruction will, I believe, be given to the pupil in the mechanisms by which this disengagement may take place, and then it will be found that the actual absorption of cultural material by the pupil will be easy and natural and the exercise of the faculties, which is now such uphill work, will be the gratifying relaxation of tensions directed to this very aim, satisfactions and fulfilments of unconscious wishes which can, with the proper understanding, be aligned with the conscious wishes.

The nearest we can come to the disengagement of the unconscious factor from the conscious in the behaviour of the pupil is to talk with him about the purposes and results of his action, and the relation between aim and achievement, to find out ourselves and show him what he is consciously striving for and the frequently opposing end which he is unconsciously attempting to gain. Analytic study of certain habits generally shows that they are attempts of the unconscious to gain satisfactions of extremely infantile desires which would be hotly repudiated by the pupil at first, but finally admitted with a salutary effect on his conduct and work.

It is very difficult not to exceed all reasonable limits in writing on a topic which opens up the unconscious element in all conscious acts. It suggests, for instance, all kinds of faulty performances, the great habitat of which is the schoolhouse, and every kind of human blunder which *habitat* everywhere. It also suggests an exposition of the modern theory of the interpretation of dreams, which are a conscious mental activity caused entirely by the unconscious thought. But as they are better classed as conscious thoughts and are not really acts, with the exception of that sporadic phenomenon of talking in one's sleep, I have mentioned them only there.*

* § 14, page 82; also see the author's *Man's Unconscious Conflict*, page 144.

Summary

The conscious and the unconscious thought and act are both identified and distinguished, and their relations discussed in detail, showing how education depends on the conscious thought being able to act as a causative factor in unconscious thought and action, and how the existence of any specific thought in the mind indicates its origin in the unconscious, from which it is thrust into consciousness by the power of the unconscious wish.

CHAPTER IV

THE PARTIAL TRENDS

THE mechanisms which are to be taken up in the next chapter are supplemented by the partial trends which differ slightly in the opposite sexes. It is customary to speak of the stream of unconscious desire as the libido or the libido trend. It should not be thought that, because this word was chosen, the libido is solely regarded as being a crassly sexual concupiscence. On the contrary the full force of the libido may, through the power of sublimation,* be directed exclusively to goals that are quite apart from the sexual. This dirigibility of the libido distinguishes the higher intellectual person from the animal-level human. It is also this capacity for sublimation which school education consciously aims at developing. As we can develop the capacity for sublimation of the individual's libido, academic education may be a success. If we could not do it, education would be a failure.

Sadism—Masochism

Some of the libido is regularly found existing in two pairs of attributes, each having opposite characteristics emanating from the active and passive form of the same trend. A tendency to inflict pain and a pleasure in

* See pages 146 and 227.

inflicting pain upon others is normally found in all healthy children at one stage in the development of their personality.   If this is not properly outgrown, or sloughed off, as are the first set of teeth or the epithelial cells of the skin, the persistence of it into the age of adulthood is an abnormality called *Sadism*.   For the Sadist the infliction of pain is essential to his own enjoyment of the pleasures of love.   This is not to say that all persons finally outgrow this tendency all at once and at a definite date.   On the contrary, most adults continue to possess a certain amount of sadistic characteristics without which it is unlikely that they would succeed wherever competition enters into the securing of any desired aim.   For a person absolutely without sadistic traits—in other words, a person in whom the inevitable sadistic traits had been completely repressed—would never take any pleasure in winning any sort of game, nor in being successful in any competition whether athletic or commercial.   He could never shoot an animal for food or hook a fish, for he would feel so keenly the suffering of the victim as to prefer to refrain from injuring him in every way.   Similarly it may be said of all the partial libido trends that they exist in both directions to a slight extent in all adults.

The partner of this trait of sadism is known as *Masochism*.   An out-and-out Masochist is one who takes the keenest pleasure not in inflicting but in suffering pain. The true masochist must suffer in order to get pleasure. As both of these traits concern pain, and the pleasure derived from inflicting and suffering it, they are called partial libido trends, and it is found that they are always paired in every individual, though in varying proportions.

And it is easy to see that if a person was preponderatingly sadistic, his masochism would be shoved into the background, and vice versa.

It is less easy to understand, though it has been shown in many analyses of both men and women, that a desire to inflict pain, deeply repressed into the unconscious, may be compensated for by a very vivid concern about other people's not suffering pain. Ardent advocates of anti-vivisectionism and of prevention of cruelty to animals and to children are quite evidently occupied mentally with the idea of cruelty. There is a great deal of creative force expended by such people on the maintenance of the idea of cruelty. For cruelty is filling their minds when they tell us so vehemently that cruelty must be stopped. The people who have no cruelty in their hearts never think of cruelty at all, and would least of all consume their nights and days in an attempt to keep other people from being cruel. It is the belief of such persons that, in order to deter, we must portray in hideous lineaments. The anti-vivisectionists have minds filled with cruelty, albeit negative cruelty. Their cruelty is not in the conscious part of their minds, but in the unconscious. They are themselves of course not aware of this unconscious content of cruelty, this repressed sadism; consciously they think themselves to be paragons of tender-heartedness. And they certainly are, if tender-heartedness is the repression of cruelty. In this case it appears, paradoxically, that the more (unconscious) cruelty, the more (conscious) kindness, and the more effusively kind a person is, the more is he compensating for unconscious sadism.

Exhibitionism

This pair of traits, consisting of the wish to hurt and to be hurt, is paralleled by the second pair, which is to see and to be seen. This appears in a noticeable degree in children but normally disappears at a certain stage of development, never again to be noticed as such, much as a bar of gold might be ground into grains and sprinkled in the sand of the sea, where it might produce but a faint lustre, or a skein of brilliant yarn, which is used as a single thread among a hundred in the weaving of a fabric.

For all children have a desire " to see and eke for to be seye." Teachers and parents well know that, while the infant has no inhibition placed on his showing his entire body or inspecting that of anyone else, much that is usefully done in later years is at least partly determined by this partial libido trend. The " exhibitionists " and " peeping Toms " of the courts are persons in whom this trait has not been broken up at the proper time before adolescence, but has persisted unchanged or amplified, a mark of undeveloped infantility.

Artists and actors are examples of the useful and productive control of this partial libido trend. The actor is rewarded by society for continuing to exhibit his body and what mentality he can, while the artist is a socially approved exhibitionist of the second degree, showing not his physical person but his spiritual qualities (his unconscious) through the medium of his art.

In the schoolroom the teacher has before him a continuous drama of only partly repressed sadism and exhibitionism, which it is his duty to ignore as far as possible and to eradicate chiefly by the substitution of interests that direct the attention of the child away from self and toward things and the relations between them.

Ambivalence

A characteristic of unconscious mentality which is based on an essential quality of the physiological structure is known as ambivalence. It roughly corresponds to opposition and antagonism, in the good senses of those terms. The body, when not comparatively relaxed as it is in sleep is maintained in any position by virtue of the opposed muscles, pairs of which in contrary tension with varying strains constantly keeping each limb in the desired position. If one of the pair should be suddenly paralysed the limb would be forcibly flexed in the other direction by the tension of the one not paralysed and the posture would come to an end.

It is quite analogous in the matter of sensations and perceptions. We have, for instance, a sensation of yellow from an orange only by virtue of the other colours which surround it. If the experiment were made of putting an orange close enough to each eye to fill the entire field of vision, we should find that the orange colour finally gave way and we had no colour sensation whatever. It may similarly be said that consciousness of any quality depends upon the constant substitution or replacement of that quality by another. The same quality cannot endure and remain conscious. With an absolute monotone dinning in our ears we finally become unconscious of tone as such, with the same odour assailing our noses unchanged we soon become oblivious of any odour.

It is interestingly and instructively analogous with regard to the emotions. These states of mind are regarded by the newer psychology more as states of matter than they have previously been regarded by the older mental science. Thus, the emotion of fear is now considered to consist of minute physical contractions of the very muscles which would be used in flight. In other words, fear is a physical preparation for flight. The importance of this fact for us in the present study is that what we consciously note in ourselves as the effects of fear or the sensation of fear is registered in the unconscious as muscle contraction and respiratory and circulatory changes which accompany actual flight. Thus, a fear, to use Frink's words,* is an " unfled flight " and anger is an " unfought fight." In suffering the emotion of fear, we are in a condition affecting not only our consciousness but our unconscious, a condition which may be described as a violent conflict between the former and the latter. It is interesting to note the contrary effects of two opposite actions of persons who are afraid. If they take active means to escape from the observed danger, the bodily sensations accompanying the emotion of fear promptly cease. The action of running is carried out externally and consciousness is absorbed in the flight. Thus the conflict which existed or might have existed between conscious reasoning about the senselessness of fear and the unconscious contraction of numerous muscles is immediately brought to an end. The individual is united body and mind. Union of body and mind always produces action. Perfect action implies union.

In the other case where fear occurs to a person who is unable to take any action the result is a conflict whose ef-

* *Morbid Fears and Compulsions,* page 254.

fects may be seen in every such case quite clearly. Such a person's limbs move convulsively, the blood leaves his face to go to his muscles where it is needed in case of their violent use, and his respiration becomes short and shallow, necessitating frequent compensation in deep sighs.

Fear, then, is flight. It is a flight that is carried out in miniature with the body in chains, so to speak, and unable to move. It is a chained man struggling to free himself from chains. In a sense, then, fear is a state of mind imposed upon us by society. Instinctively as animals we should in similar circumstances flee or attack the fancied cause of our fear, but not fear it. Society, in checking the flight or aggressiveness, has paralysed the outward, but it could not the inward, motions. Like all other veneers of society, fear is merely superficial. The agitation of the act of fear is potent witness to its not really affecting the instinctive unconscious elements of our personality.

In like manner anger is but the repressed action of fighting. Wrath is thus said to be swallowed, the expression indicating the popular and correct idea that the action is retained within the organism. Similarly hate is but retained or repressed murder, and love but an unrealized embrace. If, then, it is clearly understood how physically conditioned are all the emotions, it will be seen that a classification of them would be quite rational if based upon the types of actions which are therein internalized, so to speak. We may some day go so far as to name and classify the emotions according to the movements made in externalizing the actions which are internalized by the emotions, or even according to the muscles or groups of muscles used. (My very soul's all fist for his face.)

Realizing, then, that all emotions are but restrained activity (which is equivalent to curbed desire), one can easily see how the principle of ambivalence mentioned at the beginning of this section applies to the emotions. For not only is all motion physical and of the muscular type (possibly it would be better to say that all muscles necessarily function according to the principles of mechanics, of which the lever with its power weight and fulcrum is the fundamental type), but it all depends upon the effort and a force or object resisting it.

Thus it is easy to understand the ambivalence or dual nature of the emotions and the apparent paradoxes which they produce. Thus anger being only the suppressed form of fight, it happens very frequently that the fighters, after the fight, forget their anger and become friends again. At least that is very frequently observed with children. The actual fighting is what was desired; the muscles craved use. When this desire is satisfied, there is naturally and instinctively no motive for fighting. I am persuaded that all remaining rancour shown in civilized peoples must come from an incompleteness of the satisfaction gained in the fight on account of the fighters not letting themselves out with sufficient abandon. A real good fight is a satisfying fight and will last until idleness makes muscles fidgety.

Love and hate are similarly ambivalent toward each other. Not only does one approve and disapprove another person for qualities some of which are bad and others good, as everyone is a mixture of qualities good and bad, but one instinctively (that is, unconsciously) loves and hates the same person at the same time wholly and completely. The convertibility of the one emotion

so quickly and easily into its opposite is sufficient proof
of the fundamental ambivalence of all emotions. Furthermore, if emotions are but condensed motions, and if the
emotions must have some mental content quite as much as
movements of the body require some physical opposition,
it is quite conceivable that if the outlet for these activities
towards a person is dammed in one way, say the love way,
it will seek expression in the opposite way, particularly
if there be no middle course. And with respect to the
vehement attention necessarily given in love there can
be no other way, if love is denied, than vehement hate.
Indifference would simply mean directing the emotional
activities toward another person, who also would be the
recipient of love or hate according to circumstances.

This fact is of the greatest importance to parents and
teachers, in understanding the actions of their children and
the pupils entrusted to their care. When it is realized
by teachers that the love-hate relation indicates a high
degree of personal interest and that, with children particularly, hate can be readily changed into love, it will
be much easier for the teacher to get on with, and be loved
by, the pupil. If the child likes or dislikes the teacher
exceedingly, it is because the child particularly affects the
teacher and this affection is naturally quite ambivalent,
and according to the logical reasoning on true or false
premises may turn out either in what we call love or hate.

Ambivalence is thus clearly a fundamental attribute
of all nature, including human nature. Misconduct in the
home or disorder in the schoolroom is frequently caused
by this convertibility of conduct from one kind into its
opposite, a condition which both parent and teacher should
know, as it will remove any and all ground for resent-

ment against the children for the peccadilloes, particularly as teachers or parents usually make some inference as to the motive of the naughtiness and are themselves moved to resentment thereby.   Then, too, we now know that a strong feeling for or against a particular pupil is equally a sign of a strong interest or affection on the teacher's part.   Let no teacher say that he or she is specially troubled by such and such a boy or girl without intending to betray a greater interest in that boy or girl than the teacher consciously thinks he has.

Summary

The partial trends of the libido are the tendencies toward looking and being looked at, the active and passive phases of the same trend, and the tendency to inflict pain upon others and to enjoy the pain inflicted by others on self.   Ambivalence is the fundamental structural characteristic of all organic nature, and is seen in the interchange of opposing emotions.   Fear is described as an internally fled flight, and anger as a subjectively fought fight.

CHAPTER V

A MECHANISM is a manner in which the unconscious mentality functions and in which it influences, if it does not entirely control, the conscious life of the individual. The mechanisms are as rigidly determined by natural laws as are the physiological functions, from which indeed they are derived. The newer psychology is the first to recognize the effects of these mechanisms upon conscious life and to attempt to describe and classify them, and show their universal and constant operation upon all conscious acts and thoughts.

Old and New Psychology

In the old psychology association of ideas, attention, will, memory and discussions as to the nature of perception and the impossibility of pure sensation were the topics, and the ingenious adaptations of these concepts to concrete life were the admiration of some students and the source of a great deal of bewilderment on the part of some others. The older psychologies had next to nothing to say about sexual matters or about love. James has about one page out of the 1,400 pages of his *Principles of Psychology*. The newer psychology is practically centered on love and its different manifestations in child, adolescent and adult life. And while the older pschology was more a descriptive one, giving accounts of successive states of conscious mind, the newer psychology is a dynamic one and studies the impulses, instincts, motives and causes of thought and action, not only in consciousness but in the unconscious as well, thus taking into account a vast sphere of mental activity hitherto almost completely ignored. There were very good reasons for ignoring it, too, just because it contains a great deal of what conscious life regards as unpleasant, not to say even intolerable. But it is thought that if science is to investigate, she must have nothing closed to her. Nothing but a complete survey of what is visible will satisfy modern science, which is yet surrounded by the invisible and inscrutable. The most materialistic view does not see all, cannot explain the difference between animate and inanimate nature, no matter how completely it mechanizes thought.

It is our duty to look at as much as we can see, and look at it fearlessly. The story of the tree of knowledge of good and evil is a myth which shows a desire on the part of the people formulating it—a desire to be excused from exact knowledge, which is acquired only by painstaking effort. It is also a desire to be allowed to continue to picture in the imagination the gratification of desire, where desire can be gratified without physical effort, or without mental effort of the controlled or directed variety, but with only the spontaneous functioning of the ability to dream dreams. Science has to study the phenomena of thunderstorms as well as the theory of light, of decay as well as of growth, of disease as well as health, where indeed it finds no very sharp dividing line, and it has to study the invisible as well as the visible, the unintuitable as well as that which may be intuited, that of which we cannot have direct perception quite as much as that of which we have.

There is a psychological analogy in the questions about where, on the one hand, the child comes from, invariably asked by children either of themselves or of others, where other things come from, and where, on the other hand, ideas and emotions come from. Both depend on man's natural curiosity about the existence of things before and after they are sensed. About the existence of things we cannot see, we feel certain when we can touch them, even if they are invisible. About the existence of mental states or activities we have up to today made the same kind of judgment as we make about the existence of the flame of the candle after it is snuffed out. We know the flame is non-existent, and we have inferred, on some such analogical basis, that the mental activity, because not perceptible when, like the candle flame, it vanished from our sight, was also non-existent. As it is the duty of science to study, by means of their effects, the existence and nature of things not visible, it is also its duty to investigate things not perceptible, among which are thoughts when they are not in consciousness.

A mental image of a certain rural scene with which I am very familiar comes before my mind's eye with great vividness. At the same time I have also a sort of abridged edition of the pleasure I had when I actually saw the place twenty-five years ago. The visual image appears and disappears absolutely without my control. The same thing occurs, but with more feeling of control, with names, numbers, etc. I think I can call them up at will. The sight that has been seen even once is in the mind. It has the same existence, in every respect, as it would have if it *were* seen, only it is not seen. It is like the light waves in ether or the sound waves in air. The wind may be blowing through the bare branches of a forest and the sound waves, or undulations, or rhythms of condensation and rarefaction of the air may be there just the same, but there is no sound if there is no human ear there to translate those vibrations into sound. Just as the ear is to the air vibrations, turning them into sound, so is consciousness to the idea and turns it into a visual auditory or other image. And just as the air waves are there in the forest, or the thunderbolt in the tempest, and are not sound waves for the sole reason that there is no ear to hear them, and yet they are perfectly capable of being heard just as soon as the man or animal comes along; so the idea is in the part of the mind of which we are not conscious and exists in that unrecognized part in exactly the same form, barring only the condition that it is not cognized.

Just as we know that there is a world full of things which we cannot see, and know we cannot see either the things themselves or even pictures of them, so now in this twentieth century we know that the mental activities which enter our consciousness come into it out of a world of mental activities which each of us has in his own personality, and that this world of mental activities is as large in comparison with consciousness as is the world of all outdoors large in comparison with the confines of our own private and personal, individual indoors. Just as everything that exists in the world at the present time exists out of doors to us except what is in our own house, so everything that has ever happened within the range of our sensation exists for us in that outdoor world of our unconscious personality which surrounds and upholds the little domicile in which our consciousness is at home.   In a new sense we may say that each person lives in a world of his own isolated from every other person's world. This world is the world of his own mental activities,—at one time conscious, but now unconscious,—a world of which ordinarily he knows as little as the average person does of the earth and its different continents and oceans. As we walk on a plain the horizon is about twelve miles away from our eyes at their height of about five feet. This is a very small part of the entire surface of the earth, which is four million times as great. And if this individual does not travel there is not one chance in four million of his knowing at first hand even the existence of the rest of the earth.

About the same probability has always existed that we should ever become aware of the fact that we had any mental activity of which we are not conscious.   I am quite aware that we are unequally conscious of different things —for instance, those objects near the circumference of the field of vision we do not so clearly cognize as those right in the centre of the field.   The dimly or faintly cognized are said by some writers to be subconscious or only partly conscious.   What I refer to is the absolute non-existence in consciousness of certain ideas, and indeed most ideas for the greater part of the time, and their continuous existence in an absolutely unconscious state, but their complete existence and activity in every respect save the one exception of their not being in consciousness.

I have given (page 23) an illustration of a mental activity which was utterly unconscious, but which formed an integral part of a stream of consciousness which was very vivid.   I offer here an example of a sensation which, by the power of the unconscious wish, has been rendered imperceptible, that is, unable for a time to enter consciousness. I am looking at a table full of objects, and am looking for my box of matches which I know is there in full view, though I am unable to see it. I am conscious, in varying degree of vividness, of book or paper knife or inkstand or newspaper or what not. Yet there I stand totally unconscious of the box of matches with which I wish to light a pipe. The match box is making on my physical organism the same effect in every respect save one as if I were conscious of it. On the rods and cones of my retinae it is producing the same commotion as the wind in the forest branches with no ear there to hear it.

There is of course a cause why this match box should be concealed from my consciousness. I have injured my nerves by smoking too much and my unconscious mental activities are in a sense uniting in an attempt to make me smoke less. Does it seem that we are merely using rhetorical figures in speaking of the unconscious mental activities uniting to produce an effect? Are we merely personifying what has not a personal individuality as we personify the storm when we say it strode across the valley and climbed up the mountain side? On the contrary, we are speaking literally and not figuratively about the elements out of which the real human personality is actually made. But when I stand in front of my study table looking for, but not seeing, my box of matches, I am giving a good example of the mental state which is uncognized or unconscious, and which even so is making on the nervous system as much impression as if it were cognized or conscious.

If one state of mind can be unconscious and yet

operative, any and all others can be and probably are quite as active and quite as unconscious. In fact, modern psychology shows us that all the mental states we ever had, and possibly some we never had ourselves but inherited, are collected in the part of the mind of which we are unconscious and there, organizing themselves under the urgencies of the instincts, constitute a body of mentality to which has been given the name of the unconscious. Other proof of the causative activity of the unconscious factor of our minds is not lacking. In fact, not only is it not lacking, but it is so copious that it is a wonder it was not seen centuries before.

We began, at the outset of this section, by regarding consciousness and the unconscious as a continuum, in which it is impossible to say exactly where the one stops and the other begins, but in which there are states so profoundly unconscious that they never can be reached, so to speak, by the light of consciousness, yet they have a controlling effect on the conscious life. It is more pictorial, however, to regard the relations of the unconscious to the conscious life more as those existing between two levels of society in humanity. Take, for example, the highest which we may imagine as representing a king, and the lowest which represents a dweller in a slum in the king's capital city. The submerged tenth does wish to see and interview the king, would like in short to live on the Easy Street where the king's palace is, and, like the militant suffragettes, continually makes attempts to enter the king's presence. But there are many persons between the king and the lower level of society, effectually keeping them out from his presence.

We must imagine that there are mental activities as

much undesired by the conscious mind of every one of us as are the lower levels of society undesired by the king, and that these mental activities are kept down in the unconscious portion of our minds. If ever they come in by any chance, they are immediately thrust back, just as the man or woman of the lowest stratum of society would be hustled out of the king's presence by appointed officials, if perchance such an undesirable found entrance to the royal presence. The undesirable person is crowded back out of the royal presence. The undesirable thought is " repressed " from consciousness. Both are continuously pushing on toward the place from which they have been ejected.

Why Thoughts Push Outward

The reason that the thoughts are pushing out toward consciousness is that they are (as is all mental life) concerned with external reality; and the means for reaching external reality are the motions and activities of the body, reports of which are immediately made to consciousness by the afferent sensory nerves. The type of thoughts most concerned with eternal reality is that which would quickest change external reality into itself, and that is the use of matter for the formation of new and more individuals— in other words, the mental activity most likely to come up into consciousness is that which is concerned with reproduction of species. This is the case because the reproductive urge is the one which is the most perpetual and insistent, and it is natural that thoughts of, or based on, the action of reproduction should be the thoughts most spontaneously arising from the unconscious.

The Censor

However, as the development of human society has been such as to give in all ages and places a greater value to the performance of other acts than the instinctive act of procreation, there has sprung up universally a resistance against mere reproducing and eating. It has been universally felt that a race devoted to those two aims solely is not different from animals of lower orders in whom there is no other activity worthy of the name. But wherever the resistance against the mere following of the passions called animal has come from, it exists and has been the cause of all the strictly human phases of human life. We are not concerned here with the origin of this difference between animals and man. Here we have to do only with the fact of it and the way it is accomplished by the conscious mind. There are not plenty of conscious resistances against crass sexuality. In fact, the resistances against a purely animal life are those of consciousness primarily. The barrier set against purely animal thoughts, which continually strive to come into consciousness both in thoughts and in acts without thoughts, has been fitly compared to a censor who examines communications between people and deletes matter which is considered unsuitable for communication. So it is customary to say that the thoughts (wishes) of the unconscious which are solely concerned with material sustenance are censored. And in order to pass the censor they are disguised or costumed.

Mechanisms as Modes of Psychic Action

What causes us to see a similarity between some particular person's face and some animal's head? Or between a camel and a ship? These similarities are all very plain. The person's face and the animal's *are* alike because they possess certain features in common—two eyes (even a fish), a nose (even a cat), a mouth (even a caterpillar), and so on; and we see a likeness in the general impression because it really is there, and we can become conscious of it at once.

There are other similarities based on an identity of impressions and by most people perceived below the threshold of consciousness, but for those who have studied the impression analytically, quite consciously perceptible. A clear example of this is the quality of certain language which is called onomatopoeia, a sort of imitation, by the quality of the word, of qualities of things denoted. Such a quality of the words causes them to have a peculiar appropriateness to represent certain ideas. This poignant character of certain words when used in certain connections is due to the fact that their sound or their kinaesthetic effect while being spoken is like the sound or the feeling of the things denoted.

Much of the charm of poetry is caused by this type of imitative quality not only in the ancient languages, where in Greek,

$$\Delta\alpha\iota\mu o\nu\acute{\iota}\eta\ \alpha\epsilon\grave{\iota}\ \mu\grave{\epsilon}\nu\ \acute{o}\grave{\iota}\epsilon\alpha\iota\ o\grave{\upsilon}\delta\acute{\epsilon}\ \sigma\epsilon\ \lambda\acute{\eta}\theta\omega,$$

Daimoni | e a | ei men o | ieai ou | de se | letho

a line consisting almost entirely of vowels, very well represents the snarling voice of the enraged Zeus, or in Latin:

Atque rotis summas levibus perlabitur undas,

by its harmonies represents the very sound of the lapping of waves on the bow of the vessel, but also in English, where, for instance, Coleridge in three words puts vividly before the reader's mind the sound of the dropping of water on the deck of the marooned ship

From the sails the dew did drip,

and where Tennyson represents the sounds of a bright summer afternoon in:

The moan of doves in immemorial elms
And murmuring of innumerable bees.

In the following example from the " Ancient Mariner " the feeling of the words in the throat as they are being uttered is very like the feeling which they describe:

*With throats unslaked, with black lips baked.**

But in the psychical mechanism which I will first mention the identity is not merely a passive one of impression but is an *active* one of *behaviour*. We react to one situation as we would to another. A similarity in the environment produces a similarity in the reaction to it, more or less analogous to the similarity which the preceding illustrations show between the sound of the word and the sound of the thing denoted by the word, and which, even though an unperceived similarity for most people, produces a different reaction or attitude toward the words themselves. They have a deeper effect simply because

* Cf. Tennyson: "La*bor*ious *Ori*ent ivory, sphere in sphere."

they set in motion the unconscious perception of similarities. This unconscious perception produces a conscious result, but it is not an intellectual process when it emerges into consciousness. It is an emotional state of diffused pleasure, having as a basis the perceived similarities. This is quite in accordance with the genesis of emotions, for the majority of the emotions are of unconscious origin.

Origin of Pleasure from Similarity

We see that this must be so if we imagine how the earliest emotions in infancy connected with the self-preservative instinct took place at the time of the second feeding at the breast. The exhaustion of the nutriment absorbed in the infant's system after the first feeding produced a feeling of hunger which became one verging upon pain, and the restoring of the infant to the breast for its second meal produced a sensation in the first place of similarity as so many, if not all, of the sensations of touch, suckling, deglutition and satiety were identical with those of the first meal. The effect on the infant of this first and second experience of the world is such as to give a very strong emotional tone of pleasure to the situation of similarity in itself and to cause similarity to play a very important part in causing pleasure in after-life. There is also, in mere similarity of situation, an ease and facility of effort which creates a sense of superiority, a feeling for which the ego continually strives, so that it is not surprising to find it governing a great deal of later choice. The easy act is the one which gives the individual the greater sense of power.

In the course of development of the child's psyche there comes a time when, by virtue of the cognizance of similarity, or by analogy, the child sees the similarity between itself and other things, persons and children. It sees the likeness between a bundle of rags and a doll, between a stick and a boat, between a stone and a dock. It sees the analogy between persons and, of prime importance here, between itself and other persons. Possibly through learning the use of the words " me " and " my," it confuses these ideas and gets the notion that " what is *my* must be *me*," a very natural confusion and one common to all nations and ages, and quite parallel with the notion that there is some essential causal connection between the word and the existence of the thing it denotes.

But if " my " be " me," then my father is me, my mother is me, my dog is me, my horse is me, my pail and shovel in the ocean's sand are me, and it is but a step from that to the identification of myself with anything under heaven. The particular harm in one's thus identifying himself with other persons or with things is that one attributes the same fortune or misfortune to both. The inmate who identifies himself with Napoleon or Jesus Christ is doing nothing *different* from the child who identifies itself with its doll, but he is doing it to so extravagant a degree that we make him an inmate.

Identification

The mechanism called *identification*, based on similarity, is an unconscious mental process which underlies a great deal of conscious thinking and acting. One identifies oneself with other persons and things in such a way that those persons or things are regarded as a part of oneself. Indeed it is, when we consider it closely, a difficult problem to decide where the average person conceives his ego to end and the external world to begin. Physically our digestion identifies our food with our bodies literally. Mentally we regard certain parts of ourselves as more intimately ourselves than other parts. For example the attached parts of our finger nails are more closely a part of us than are the unattached parts which we cut off from time to time and our hair is not so intimately a part of ourselves as our eyelashes. Furthermore, some of our possessions we identify with ourselves much more than we do others. A pocket-knife or a purse, one suit of clothes or another, or in the case of a wealthy man one of his residences may, to use a purely figurative expression, " contain more of him " than another. He has " put more of himself into " one place than another. And so on with all the things with which we have any relation whatever. Many persons have written lists of the ten or a hundred " best books," which are only expressions of identifications which they have made between themselves and the books.

From our earliest years we identify ourselves with persons. In our desires, both conscious and unconscious, we identify ourselves on the one hand with our fathers and on the other with our mothers. Later there is a perfectly normal identification in the love we feel toward our life partners. A curious and important fact not generally known is that when at a later date we have ceased to identify ourselves with our parents as they are at present, we still retain in the unconscious the original identification which we formed at an early date with the parent as he or she then was. A man, for instance, who at the age of five years or earlier identified himself with his father, and felt like him in every respect in which he knew him and strove to imitate him in all ways, will, at the age of forty, still maintain in his unconscious a tendency to make his identification with all men who resembled in the slightest degree what his father was thirty-five years before.

In one man * who had a very stern, strict and aggressive father and identified himself with this early form in which his father existed for him even to the extent of acting both as aggressive father in his desires and compliant submissive environment in his acts, repeated the compliant submissive element of that combination whenever he met a man who resembled his father in being aggressive. He would, when caught unawares, say " Yes, sir! " to a gruff waiter, or meekly obey a car conductor uncivilly yelling to the passengers to " move forward." All the time, however, he was repeating the aggressive element in his idea of what a man should be, and, wherever not himself intimidated, was acting in an overbearing manner toward others, thus in both ways repeating the total pattern of behaviour at the age of forty, a pattern which his soul had had stamped on it at the age of five or under, by the particular father whom he happened to have and whom he came to know through the experiences which he then had of him.

Depth of Very Early Impressions

If these early impressions are so very formative, and so very lasting, it becomes at once evident that they must

* Frink: *Morbid Fears and Compulsions,* p. 212.

be reformed as early in the child's life as possible. It has not been found possible to do much in the way of influencing the individual's unconscious *before* the age of puberty, except through the parents. In this case it is really the parents who should be educated, for they alone by their actions can cause the early impressions of their children, so important for their later welfare, to be wholesome and normal and prevent the damage which is inflicted then and does not have its full force sometimes for over a quarter of a century.

Education which should affect this very vital part of the individual's life should of course be directed to the child's entire environment from the earliest days of its existence. As it is at present quite impossible adequately to control this, the problem for education, if education is to be thorough and penetrating, is to take the child, spiritually maimed in many cases by its early environment, and reshape it during school and college days in such a way as to remove the multitude of wrong impressions which are inevitable now with most children and which affect the working of the mechanisms of which I have already mentioned only identification, the others being much less simple and much more subtle in their influence on the conscious life.*

Primary Identifications

It should not be omitted here that the most universal identification is that of the boy with his mother (and that of the girl with her father), an identification which, being of opposite sex, has an effect not only upon the

* This will be taken up in greater detail in the next chapter.

individual's choice of a love mate but also on the way in which he or she behaves to the mate. If the husband identifies himself with his mother he will identify himself in exactly the same way with his wife, and there then results in his psyche an objective identification of the two persons, mother and wife. When, therefore, a husband behaves toward his wife as a child should toward its mother, expecting from the wife in all ways exactly the kind of tenderness which he originally received from his mother, he fails to act in every respect as a man should act toward his wife. The same statement can be made, *mutatis mutandis*, about the attitude of the wife toward her husband, determined as it is by her identification, first of herself with her father and with her husband and then of her father and her husband.

Identifications in School

It may be asked at this point what can be done by the teacher in school to correct the undesirable element in these identifications. In college the faculty adviser can of course go specifically into the details of this and the other mechanisms, but in school that will of course be impossible. But the teacher, if made aware of this simple mechanism, can act toward the pupils in such a way as to train them away unconsciously, in a small degree to be sure, from the excesses of this identification and principally by means of inducing them to become as independent in their work as possible. Children tend to identify a woman teacher with the mother and to seek from her the sympathy and help which they early received from their mothers, and a teacher, with the laudable desire of being loved, will tend, unless she realizes the weakness which she is perpetuating in her wards, to over-accentuate the helpfulness which is so highly appreciated by the pupil.

The earliest task imposed upon the child in school should therefore be that which he can accomplish by his own unaided efforts.   The identification of the task with the teacher is almost universal and is the initial mistake. This identification takes place in several ways.   It is seen in the very common phenomenon already mentioned that the task is accomplished *for* the teacher, and the chief pleasure and reward for the child comes from the praise and affection bestowed by her on the pupil, and, more important still, the fact that the child likes and does well in those studies where the teacher is personally attractive to the child.   Here the task is identified with the teacher in the most concrete form, and it is clear that the elements in the child's performance which should make for his independence are reduced almost to nothing and its educative force almost annihilated in proportion to the extent of the identification.   The first effort of the teacher should therefore be to change the attitude of the child toward the task and encourage his independent activity toward the world of reality, the only taste of which procurable within the cloister of the school is the feeling on the part of the child that he is mastering a part of something which is external to himself.   This will not be the case if he identifies the task with the teacher.

In this connection it is an unfortunate fact that the early tasks of the school are generally those in which he is almost unable to express any individuality different from other children's.   When, for instance, the same ten examples in arithmetic are given to a class of forty children, and the forty sets of answers have to be exactly the same for each child, there is little scope for individuality. If the child wishes to be individual and make his work his own and different from other children's he must have different answers to the examples—answers which are called *wrong!* The effect is no less undesirable, even though it be inevitable, just as any lock step is undesirable, though it be the only or the easiest means of accomplishing what seems to be the purpose of public education. From this point of view we see identification in another of its aspects, the identification of the pupils each with the other, a form of this mechanism which is seen at its highest degree of development in a flock of sheep.

From the teacher's own point of view identification of the objective kind is of the greatest importance, as it unconsciously makes him identify the pupils with each other, and prevents him from regarding them as individualities themselves.   It is unlikely that the teacher will be able to correct his own defective attitude toward his pupils if he is unacquainted with this mechanism and its operation in his own unconscious thoughts and acts. Identification is the easiest method of mental procedure. It becomes automatic and gives the greatest feeling of power because it seems to enable him to handle forty persons as one.   In identification the similarities are selected and emphasized and the differences are ignored, no matter what may be their real practical importance.   When the teacher realizes that identification is one of the main modes of unconscious thought and not only that it is operative in his pupils but also in a large measure in himself and in all other teachers, he will better understand

what his own specific problems are with regard to the part
he is to play in the education of the young.

He will all the more keenly feel the necessity of an
individual study of his pupils and will be enabled to make
the greater allowance for his own actions and *theirs*.
He will realize that, while a certain amount of identification is necessary in all human thinking, in the formation
of abstract ideas, he is by virtue of his knowledge of
analytic psychology in a position to measure the amount
of identification in himself and in other teachers and adjust
his own actions accordingly. To what extent does he
identify his pupils with each other? How much dis-
tinctive individuality does each possess for him? How
far does he allow the pupils to identify with himself the
subject-matter which he teaches, and how intensively
does he strive to develop to the best of his ability the
pupils' independence of himself, of the school, of their
parents?

Two varieties of identification of the individuality with
externals are known as projection and introjection, projection being known as objective and introjection as subjective identification. The commonest form of this
mechanism is the projection of a reproach. Frequently
it is the only explanation of certain forms of suspicion.
All children and many adults act as if they believed that
others knew what was going on in their own minds.*

Projection

If a child has done something for which it feels guilty,
it will be very difficult for it not to show some sign that it

* Cf. p. 124.

feels conscience-smitten, and it will itself be filled with the feeling that other people must know something about the mischief and blame it just as it blames itself. Conscience therefore, which is the voice of their fathers and mothers heard in reality in earlier days, but now heard in imagination, forces them to think that other people are blaming them, when it is really their own consciences that are accusing them. In such a case there is an identification between the personality of the child and the personality of the other person. It is called an objective identification because the thoughts which originate solely in the child's mind are attributed to another's mind. Of this the child is unconscious, and the result is a self-deception on the child's part. If we should call the child the subject and the other person the object, then this form of identification is called objective for the reason that the mind state is attributed by the subject *to the object.*

It is an everyday occurrence and regularly unconscious in the majority of people. It is almost impossible for some people to free themselves from this form of irrationality, but the less people are governed by reason and the more by emotion, the more difficult it is to prevent this form of identification. It is quite true, too, that a certain amount of identification of the objective kind is of great social value, as it is the basis for true sympathy, and for a great many of the finer sentiments of love. A mother identifies herself with her children and is pained with them and rejoices with them. The identification of mother and daughter is given poetical expression in the beautiful and familiar passages from the Book of Ruth.

Introjection

If the feelings and thoughts of the subject are identified by the subject with those of the object, we call it objective identification or projection. If, on the other hand, the feelings and thoughts or other circumstances of some other person are objectively and definitely pictured and are identified by the subject with the subject's own mind-states or other conditions, then we have introjection or subjective identification.

This is exemplified familiarly by the state of mind many people acquire while reading books or articles about diseases. Having gained an idea from the book or magazine about the symptoms of the disease, they introject it into themselves. Projection would work the other way. They would then, if they had some uneasiness themselves, instinctively imagine that everyone else had the same. It will be seen that introjection is a sort of imitation, in causing an individual to change so as to be like a model which has been held up to him. Thus biographies and histories are useful means for an advantageous employment of the natural trend toward subjective identification or introjection. It might be said that this unconscious mechanism is the basis on which is set all the academic education of a formative or cultural type, and is the major premise on which the entire educational syllogism rests. If we teach geometry, it is with the implication that the clearness and accuracy and finality of its theorems will be introjected into the mind of the pupil. When we give the pupils literary masterpieces to read, it is with this idea alone, that the excellences of the literature in form and matter may be introjected into the mind of the pupil. And it is so introjected, and the effect of the process is complete and total, the only difficulty being that while the introjection inevitably takes place, its effects are not at once perceptible to teacher and parent. An immediate projection is naïvely expected by educators in the form of a mental expression which shall show the instantaneous impress of the form of the literary masterpiece. In the composition or essay the state of mind of the pupil should be projected upon some external object, say the air or the paper; and should show all the qualities that have been introjected by the teacher from the masterpiece. This might be regarded by the most rational as a prodigious projection on the part of the educator, and I have seen not a few teachers who attribute to the pupil a great deal of the academic mental viewpoint which teachers themselves have, and are as unsettled by their subsequent recognition of the discrepancy between their insulated views and the actual conditions as is any neurotic by his occasional actual contact with the world of reality.

We give the pupil Latin to learn partly so that he may the better understand the structure of English, which is fifty per cent fossilized Latin. We try to show him the pretty shapes formed by the fossils. Partly, however, we believe that a successful introjection can be effected through which the thought-forms of the ancient Romans may be assimilated by the modern American boy or girl, and the structure of their cogitations much strengthened. As we ourselves do in reading a book or a magazine article about diseases, we expect the student to do, in getting the ideas as they exist in external reality and subjectively identify a goodly number of them with his own mental states, and show us immediately the effect on him so that we teachers who are standing impatiently by, with tapes and rulers, may take a measure of the effects we have produced on him. When, however, we fully realize what a long-winded and difficult proposition it is for a trained psychologist to discover and modify any of the mechanisms of the unconscious, we shall appreciate how ridiculous are 'some of the expectations of the educator.

But to return to a serious consideration of the difference between projection and introjection. We have seen that projection is the attributing of an external origin to that which was really only a mental state. This does not imply always that the person so projecting is in any way abnormal. We all do it, and do it daily. Much that we see is only in our own minds, and in general we do not err in attributing it to external reality, for though it is not really there it is as good as there because it is there as far as we are concerned. This is true of a great many of the qualities attributed to music, art and literature, it is true of a great many qualities which we attribute to persons we love or admire, and the actual non-existence of the qualities as an objective reality is not only of no moment, but our unconscious self-deception in this line is of value to us in making the world livable. But it is only when the qualities which we attribute to external persons or things are disproportionately exaggerated that we come to grief. Then projection becomes a disease itself and requires heroic measures if it is to be cured.

It has been said that projection is a mechanism by which the individual psyche defends itself against the unpleasant situations of life and originates at the time when the infant first makes a distinction between himself and the external world. There is inaugurated at that time a mental connection between things that cause pain or discomfort and external objects. Things which are unpleasant are in a sense rejected by the unconscious mind of the child, and because they are thus rejected are considered as not a part of the self but a part of what is opposed to the self—a part, in other words, of the real externality which makes bumps and hurts of various kinds. Thus when at a later date the individual is led by his unconscious to do something instinctive which society disapproves and he is mildly or severely condemned by society, or by his conscience the representative of society in his own soul, he as instinctively tends to project the whole incident and regard the act not as his own but as another's.

It is even more so with thoughts. Every person has thoughts which emanate from the unconscious and are the conscious forms of unconscious desires. Those thoughts, if they appear in the form of criticisms of his own conduct, which is a very common way for them to appear, are cast, so to speak, in the character of someone else—someone, for instance, who would be likely to criticize the action in question, or who the individual supposes would be likely to do so. If a person feels that someone else would criticize or blame him for doing some act—such, for instance, as riding on a public conveyance without paying fare, or taking an undue proportion of profit in the sale of merchandise—it is ten to one that the criticism is more subjective than objective. Of course any sensitive and high-strung individual is likely to do that, and it is only when the thing becomes excessive, and interferes with other activities that it becomes abnormal. The absolutely matter-of-fact person does not in these circumstances have the idea of criticism or blame occur to him in this connection. The mere fact that the idea occurs is enough to prove that it is of subjective origin, and not a true experience from the outside world, contributed by someone else. In the case where a degree of censure falls upon a person not showing this projection mechanism, such person reacts in a totally different way. He stoutly denies the existence or the importance of the act or its significance, or if it be merely a thought that occurs to him, he dismisses it as mere nonsense and is not troubled by it further. But, in the person with a tendency to project reproaches, the criticism is falling on a very receptive soil and takes root and thrives, and as the individual is not acquainted wth the idea that many reproaches are solely of internal origin, he thinks that other people may be thinking ill of him.

Mechanism of Blame *

Perhaps here would be an appropriate place to indicate some of the corollaries deducible from this principle with regard to the placing of blame, to the utterance of censorious criticism, and to the question of punishment. Believing that an error is but the miscarrying of a wish to create, one cannot consistently attribute blame to anyone, man, woman or child, nor say that any act is a fault. Entirely aside from the very important psychological consideration that the attributing of blame to

* This illustrates the projection of a reproach, mentioned page 118.

anyone is concentrating the attention on the destructive aspect of his act, magnifying it in a way particularly gratifying to him, and satisfying in an ill-advised way his desire for personal attention, blaming anyone for what he has done once or habitually does is a very irrational procedure for a teacher who believes that many acts are caused by unconscious thoughts, for the reason that no person who has not been introduced to his own unconscious and shown a method of controlling it, can be held responsible for what it makes him do. This fact does not of course release a pupil from real responsibility for his conscious acts done from conscious thoughts. It only places the responsibility for certain errors of performance where such responsibility really belongs, if causation by the unconscious thoughts can be said to involve any responsibility.

Thus a woman teacher would not be likely to feel any real resentment toward an adolescent boy for any misdemeanour if she realized that his disorder was really prompted by love of herself, by a desire, unconscious on his part, to be sure, to have her attention, to have her look at and talk to him. If she knew enough about unconscious mental mechanisms to realize *that,* she would not blame him, but would be able to use that unconscious affection for her for the purpose of getting him to transfer his creative desires to things of the external world more appropriate to his own development than herself. If, on the other hand, she responds to his unconscious love-making, and attends to his " faults " and not to the work which he ought to be doing, she is herself guided unwittingly by her own unconscious. For her interest in him, even her irritation, is an expression of her own unconscious wish to attract him. The more he can irritate her—and his unconscious is prompting him to do it as intensively as possible, for his unconscious is unwittingly attracted to her personality—the more will the situation be a personal one which approaches real love-making as its limit, and forgets or ignores the true purpose which brought them together. Of course the child is not supposed to know this, and the teacher does not always know it either, though from the time when the unconscious is recognized as a factor in education she will know it, and logically pursue a true educational aim, cease to be irritated and get real happiness out of the situation.

Separation of Self from World

As the infant begins its mental life with an innate identification of itself with the external world, the first thing it learns is that a part of this " self," as we might call the sum total of infantile experience, is independent of that part of the world which is most its personal subjective self, and is not under its control. This is equivalent to saying that a separation has to take place between the individual and the world as the first step in its education. The resolution of this primary identification continues and forms one of the important aims of academic education in the earlier years. At the same time there is a secondary separation from the world, after the child makes the original separation, and learns the difference between itself and external reality. This secondary separation follows the finding out that things cannot always be controlled, but that generally thoughts can, and consists in a retreat into self, a flight from reality, which unfits the individual for true wholesome adult contact with it quite as much as would the maintenance of the original infantile identification.

The teacher has under his observation less of the first separation from the world than has the parent, for most of it takes place before the child comes to school, though not all. But during the later grammar grades and in the high school the secondary separation, or segregation, tends to take place and has constantly to be combated both by teacher and parent, so that the final aim is in a sense the reverse of the initial aim of education, namely, to unite the individual with the world from which under certain circumstances he tends more and more to separate himself. Complete education, therefore, regarded solely from the point of view of the individual's relation to the world of external reality, forms a cycle in which the individual is first separated from the world and then united with it, and in a sense separated from himself. This is accomplished by giving the thoughts and acts as external a reference as possible.

Identification with Work

This externalization of the thoughts and acts may take place in every hour of every school day, or, from some technical error in school management, it may fail to take place. The pupil should be taught so to throw himself into the work as, in a certain sense, to identify himself with it. He should be taught that a complete absorption in work, while he is at work, will enable him to be completely absorbed in play, when playtime comes around. Lest it be inferred that I am here favouring a strenuosity of life which ill accords with the nervous natures of some pupils, I say that there should be some, if even a very little, time devoted to day-dreaming, provided the pupil knows what he is doing and how different in character it is from true thinking directed toward a definite goal. And it should not be inferred either that a programme can be made out, with a time-table, showing just so much directed thinking, so much play and so much day-dreaming, at times which are at the same hour and of the same length for all pupils of the same grade. For the programme and the time-table are as impossible, in the highest development of personality, as are the uniform size and positions of school furniture.

In order to develop the individual to his highest degree of personality, it will eventually have to come to individual methods in education. The teacher will have to know human nature so thoroughly, a knowledge which can be acquired only through a knowledge of the unconscious as well as of conscious life, that if he has more than one pupil he may be able to get at the root of any difficulties they may have in a time much shorter than he devotes to a whole class at the present time. His words will have to be few but telling. A class of twenty-five with recitations of forty-five minutes each week for twenty weeks a term would give each child a whole week a term of individual instruction. How much could be told each child in that time, even by the most skilful teacher, provided that instruction were the aim and not education? How much could a child learn from a teacher in 225 minutes a term? Certainly to improve the quality of the work the teacher does for the child, a great improvement is necessary in the skill of the teacher. And of course the average child does not get 225 minutes a term, 450 minutes a year, from the teacher, because the classes are larger and the weeks are fewer in most schools.

But if it could be proved that all the *good* the child gets from the teacher is received only in the times of personal, individual contact which he does get, say about three minutes a day, it would seem quite worth while to change things so that he could get more. That is, provided the teacher was so constituted as to be worth it. If as taxpayers we could see that more individual attention of teacher to pupil was fully worth all that was expended for it, it would be cheap at any price, which proves that as taxpayers we do not believe it. In other words, we believe that what the child gets in school he gets more from the building and from the other children and from his own efforts than he does from the teacher. But what a very unbusinesslike proposition that is! As well say that physicians could cure their patients in classes of thirty in a magnificent hospital building by hearing them recite their symptoms and telling them what to do and not to do.

Individual Attention to Pupil

And all the more is it necessary to give the children a greater amount of special attention and pay the teachers more liberally to enable them to give it, when it is realized that the problem in teaching is not alone the subject-matter of instruction and not alone the conscious thought of the child about the subject, but, more necessary than all that, is the teacher's knowledge of the unconscious thoughts his own and the pupil's. This is an entirely new science which the teacher of the near future will have to have, and be more proficient in, than in the " subject " which he is supposed to know. Teachers are now examined in the theory of education, and to a certain extent in psychology, before they are granted licenses to teach. But the newer psychology, as applied to education, is something that soon will be demanded of every competent teacher.

It is not to be denied that a few "born teachers " have instinctively grasped the main principles of the newer psychology, and their work in the classroom is as good as a knowledge of the newer psychology could make it, but they are very few indeed. The state should take it upon itself to see that the work of all teachers is as good as that of the " born teacher." This cannot be done without a knowledge of the working of the unconscious part of the mind.

Compensation

Any paired organ of the body naturally extends its activities or sharpens its abilities if the other of the pair is damaged or destroyed. Thus, one eye being injured, the other frequently takes an added responsibility and does the work for two. One may even regard the different senses as paired in this connection. A person becoming blind gains greater acuity of hearing or greater sensitiveness of touch.

This is exactly what takes place in those faculties

which we call mental but which, being based on the physical properties of matter, ought rather to be called material-mental or psycho-physical. Automatic adjustments take place all over the body all the time, apparently designed by nature to adapt the organism to the changing circumstances of its environment. Thus the approach of danger sensed by the unconscious produces many changes in the body of which consciousness is not aware. It sends an increased amount of sugar to the muscles, a substance which they consume in greater amount in more strenuous physical exertion. It aërates the blood by producing a more rapid respiration, and to the blood it furnishes also a principle which makes it much more likely to clot in case of a wound.

Analogous to these physical preparations which go on in the body below the level of consciousness, there are many mental processes which take place below the threshold of consciousness. This is not to say that these mental processes take place as preliminaries to an emotion after which the emotion ensues, but it is nearer the truth to say that these processes *are* the emotion, and that part of the emotion of which we are conscious is but the effect of these unconscious mental processes upon the consciousness itself.

What then, it may be asked, is the advantage gained by calling these processes mental, and in what way are they to be distinguished from physical processes? In answer it may be said that the distinction between mental and physical processes is a philosophical problem which is irrelevant to a chapter on psychology and still more so in a book on the application to educational problems of the hypotheses of a new type of psychology.

A word should be said here about the deterministic implications which will by some people be attributed to this mode of thinking. If our thoughts, as seems to be implied, are the effects of processes (whether mental or physical) which take place apart from consciousness and according to the laws of the physical world as studied by natural science, what hope is there that the individual is now, or ever will be, able to have a will free enough to control not physical matter, but even the coming and going and selection of his own thoughts? This is a topic which has been discussed for ages and belongs rather in a metaphysical treatise than in a psychological one. In this book I am attempting only an exposition of the principles of the newer psychology, an exposition which I hope will put some of our educational problems in a new light for other teachers as it has done for me.

The physiological processes go on all the time in the body without coming into consciousness and being recognized for what they are. Undoubtedly they do produce a remote effect upon conscious mental states. We are all familiar with them. The presence in the stomach of ill-chewed, rapidly swallowed, inadequately salivated food causes at times a form of indigestion to which is attributed as an effect an emotional state appropriately called sourness of temper. Yet we do not call the sourness of temper or any of the feelings or acts which it evokes and which are admittedly consciously perceived—we do not call these the perception of the indigestion. What is it that is felt? As well ask what is it that is seen when we look at a plum pudding. Do we see a white dish, with a brown and black mass on it, over which hovers a pale blue vapour? Strictly speaking, we do not perceive any of those things until after we have learned what they are.

Nor do we perceive either the unconscious or any of its effects as such until we learn what it is and what they are. The method of discovery and the nature of the inference by which the existence and qualities of the unconscious are deduced or inductively inferred is a matter of the deepest interest, but can only be touched upon here. It is somewhat similar to the mental processes by which the planet Neptune was first supposed by astronomers to exist, though invisible, and later seen in the calculated position when the telescopes of higher power were made.

From the aberrant behaviour of certain planets the attraction of a larger, remoter invisible body was inferred. *From mental aberrations* of our conscious states has been deduced the existence of the larger, and in a sense remoter, imperceptible psychic entity in the personality of each and every one of us. That is, the thoughts and actions are called aberrant, just as the motions of the planets were, until the presence of the larger body was known. Then they were recognized (cognized again) as not in the least aberrant. They did not depart from the laws of motion. Therefore what astronomers did when they found that the so-called irregularities of the planets' motions were not irregularities at all, except from a narrow point of view, was exactly what psychologists are now doing when they discover that what have been called mental aberrations are not departures from natural law, but are illustrations of it. They were the working of a cause which had not yet been discovered or traced to its ultimate principle. For instance, many of the acts of insane persons have been attributed by the newer psychology to the fact that the insane are in a great many senses merely children of a larger growth and their actions are determined by a persisting infantility.

The purpose of this long disquisition on these aspects of the theory of the unconscious is to lay the foundation for an understanding and insight into the mechanisms of thought as they have been revealed by the more modern type of psychological research.

We have seen so far that ambivalence is that mental attribute which corresponds to the antagonism of forces in the purely physical realm, and is seen in the psychic sphere in such traits of general nature as the existence of love and hate *in* the same person *for* the person, at the same time, being thus an attribute of the emotional life. And we have just begun to discuss the attribute of compensation which we saw clearly exemplified in the physiological sphere in several types of action.

A compensation is a conscious effect of an unconscious cause. Why not, then, call it merely an effect and not put another name to it? For the reason that in the concept of compensation the effect is regarded as analogous to its cause and not of an entirely different classification. This analogy includes direct contraries. As is seen in the section on ambivalence (page 93), a strong desire for a certain person expressed in love will be turned instantly into hate, both of which enter consciousness, sometimes to the utter surprise of the person concerned. An old proverb says that a woman who hates a man either has loved, does love or will love him. In a compensation, however, only one member of the analogy enters consciousness, while ambivalence keeps both members of the equation, both sides of the balance, so to speak, *below* the threshold of consciousness. It is only in the mechanism of compensation that one of the pair of activities appears in consciousness. A person will compensate with conscious actions for an unconscious desire, just as he will balance two conscious desires and throw more impetus into the one because it is a socially approved one, for the reason that he has already thrown more than he thinks he ought into the other, and he wishes to keep a certain balance between what he instinctively wants to do and what, from his experience of society, he thinks *it* wants him to do. By keeping an even balance in this way he satisfies his conscience and does not worry.

A corollary of this compensating for an unconscious desire by means of a conscious one is that we have no conscious desires that are not compensations. It is quite evident that as the unconscious desires are the pressure of the animal instincts, against which society has set up numerous barriers, we should, if we followed these all the time, do practically nothing of all the complicated web of human activities which now we are weaving. If no barriers of society whatever opposed us, we should have no compensatory mechanisms such as we now have. There would be no restraint or repression. But the moment we have any restraint opposed against us, we attempt to fulfil our desires in some other way, provided we cannot overcome the restraint. If a runaway, or a river, comes to a wall or a dam, he goes over it or around it if he cannot knock it down. The going around it is the compensation for the going over, which he (or it) cannot do.

Substitution

Thus through compensation, which means quite as much libido directed against another object when it is obstructed by one object, we necessarily make use of substitutes. In other words, a strong desire is for some definite thing, unless it is for promiscuous muscular activity, and then kicking or running or swimming will satisfy. But it is a familiar human experience that when we want any specific thing it is possible to transfer that desire to some other thing. In this case we do not so much compensate as substitute. Generally a compensatory mechanism is a reaction in consciousness to an unconscious stimulus, while a substitution is the replacement of one thought or act in consciousness by another thought or act in consciousness. Furthermore the term compensation is more extensive; that is, a long and complicated course of action may be called a compensation mechanism, while a single idea or mannerism of action—in other words, a small unit of activity—is likely to be called a substitute formation.

Both compensations and substitutions are mediated through mere displacements of ideas. One idea displaces another in the mind and one idea is substituted for another idea as the goal-idea of a desire. This is not the same as saying that one idea follows another in the mind, each idea giving way before, and in that sense being displaced by, its successor. That would be a purely descriptive statement of what actually takes place in the mind because our stream of consciousness is never other than one idea following another. But a displacement or a substitution is an idea which takes the place of another idea in the mind at all times when that second idea, which we might call the original idea, would naturally (that is, if there were no repressions) appear in the mind. The original idea is a banished idea, not allowed to enter consciousness, and, as if it had a desire of its own to enter consciousness which it could satisfy vicariously, it sends its representative or proxy to act for it. Thus in displacement is implied an inability of the idea which is displaced to enter consciousness, together with its being unknown for what it really is and frequently there is implied a power of the displaced, covered, shrouded, masked idea to work, in the unconscious, physical ill on the individual for whom it is a masked idea, due no doubt to the individual's consequent inability to adjust it to the remainder of his personality, which as he cannot see it, he is unable to do.

While one idea may be substituted for another as the goal idea of a desire, the desire remains the same, not in content but in strength. Heine said that the French put as much energy into their pursuit of liberty as ardour into the affection for their chosen brides, while the Germans look upon liberty as they do upon their aged grandmothers. A man may devote his entire energy, which means his entire libido, to an abstract cause, or he may consume it in the love of a fair mistress. He may also, if the fair lady has rejected him, and he finds no physical outlet for his excited emotions, spend them upon himself.

Displacement

In identification and compensation we have seen a conscious thought displacing, or substituted for, an unconscious desire. Displacement is the generic term describing these substitutions of conscious thought and action for the natural instinctive unconscious thoughts which, though continuously pushing forward toward consciousness, are transformed in such a way that they are acceptable to the social conventions of conscious life. The thought and action of which we are conscious in ourselves and in others is invariably a displacement, a disguise under which the unconscious wish passes the censor and enters consciousness, a disguise without which it would be opposed. Only those thoughts and actions which are vigorously opposed as immoral when they enter consciousness, as they do occasionally as crime, heresy, etc., are the natural and undisguised unconscious wishes.

The classroom actions of the pupil are disguised or substituted actions in almost every case. And we are constantly requiring the pupil to make substitutions in his own action for the actions which his unconscious wishes would cause him to perform. In a sense that is what school and education are for. But we reason that a superimposed substitution will have the same good result as a naturally developed one. Here is an instance:

It is quite true that a middle-aged man may sit gladly for hours (but not every man, at that) with a pen in his hand writing in a book, and an almost infinitesimal proportion of men will write books which will have an influence on the acts of their fellow-men. But to think that the influential words are caused by the sitting still is an evident fallacy, and yet that is exactly what we are doing in schools everywhere. The position in which we put the pupil is analogous to that of the middle-aged writer, before a desk and holding a pen, and the reasoning is exactly that of the savage who makes an image of his conception of a god and puts food before it. The savage thinks: This image will eat this food and be pleased with me and grant me a favour, exactly as I was pleased and did a favour for someone who set food before me.

We seem to have reasoned the same way. Just as good may come from a mature man sitting at a desk, so will good come from the immature man sitting at a desk. And this is a mental displacement (identification) just as erroneous, but just as dynamic psychologically because *it has produced* the present classroom requirements, as is the identification which the pupil makes of the teacher with the stern father or mother, or which the teacher makes of the pupil in identifying him with a previously experienced disorderly one. Similarly when a nervous woman comes to a physician for treatment and one of the symptoms is an exaggerated solicitude for her mother or her children we have another displacement. Like all unconscious displacements it is the substitution of one idea for another. In the case of the nervous woman she replaced desire which was in her unconscious with its opposite, anxiety, in her conscious life, and by the strength of her solicitude she expressed the real depth of her unconscious desire that her mother should die. By the sternness with which we repress the movements of the child do we similarly express the depth of our unconscious desire to let him give full play to his instincts and develop them in a rational manner. The exaggerated concern of a daughter for her mother's health or of a mother for that of her children has frequently been found to be a conscious over-compensation for the opposite wish in the unconscious. I think our present insistence upon uniformity and silence and motionlessness on the part of the school child is similarly an over-compensation for our real unconscious feeling that they need to move more than they do. And of course the thing works out in the opposite direction. The child over-compensates for his unconscious desire to neglect lessons by an occasional over-vigorous spurt of accomplishment.

It may be said that a noticeably strong conscious tendency in any direction is likely to indicate the presence of an opposite tendency in the unconscious, much as a convexity on one side of a thin metal plate corresponds to a concavity on the other side. And in each case it is really the same force which produces the unevenness. Any unevenness in character, or idiosyncrasy or eccentricity is thus seen to be the work of unconscious forces, the conscious form in which they are displayed almost invariably being a displacement of some sort.

Here we have reasoning by analogy carried out in a psychological and not a logical manner, and commit all the blunders which can be committed in so doing. Displacement is technically defined as the using of the wrong ideas with the wrong emotions, or vice versa, the psychical putting of things in the wrong place. When the displacement reaches an extreme, as it does in cases which psychiatry calls anxiety hysteria, the emotions which properly belong to certain ideas are taken away from those ideas entirely. The ideas are themselves repressed into the unconscious, but the emotions, which cannot be repressed, are attached to other ideas which in normal persons are not associated with such strong emotions.

If, for instance, a person is excessively afraid of snakes or of thunderstorms or of tunnels or of dogs or what not, and has a fear of them which other persons ridicule and which neither they nor the timorous person can account for, then they exemplify this displacement between idea and emotion. Similarly any complete inability on the part of any pupil to master a given task may be caused by a similar displacement. The emotions which are engendered by the task are quite disproportionate to it. Therefore they belong not to it but to some other idea which, if the teacher knows enough, may be discovered and the excessive emotion may be disengaged from the task in question.

I do not mean to say that there should be no emotion, no excitement, no liveliness in the schoolroom. All of these are necessary, both on the part of the pupil and of the teacher. In the pupils the emotions are properly expressed in activity which necessarily results in noise in the undraped room. I refer only to the type of emotion which is appropriate and which is seen in all schoolrooms where real honest effort is being made. There is no objection to frequent bursts of laughter, if they are the result of the pupils' perception of relations of the subject-matter, and not mere deriding the unsuccessful efforts of some supposedly stupid pupil. Of course it is unfortunate that we have not yet arrived at the state of civilization where the physical activities can be more gradually tapered off and the sublimation of physical into mental energy is not authoritatively demanded at once.

I know a high school, for instance, where the first experience of the incoming student is being required to sit for two hours and a half in the assembly hall, where absolute silence and motionlessness is sternly demanded, and the unfortunate child who forgets and talks to his neighbour is required to take a seat on the platform and be eyed by a thousand children as an example. I know of no house of public entertainment where people gladly pay money for a seat, in which the performance of two and a half hours is not broken three or four times and the audience is given an opportunity to relax. But in our present school system, so powerfully are we dominated by the silence of the printed page that we act as if we supposed that directed thinking could be immediately produced by suppression of the physical expression of the undirected variety, all the motions of most children belonging in this class.

In adult human life many of the most intensely interested persons are intense in certain directions by virtue of a displacement of over-compensation. Antivivisectionists frequently by their activity show an over-compensation for unconscious desire to inflict cruelty, the significant fact being that whether they were consciously or unconsciously cruel, they would be equally concerned psychically with the idea of cruelty, an idea which, to the ordinary person, has been outgrown with the other infantile attributes. Militant feminists, when women, are frequently giving expression by their excessive militancy to an unconscious wish not to rule and be the equals of men but to be ruled and dominated by *a man*. Lynching is another expression in consciousness of an unconscious desire for cruelty. Few members of a lynching party, if interrogated, would admit that they took pleasure in the sufferings of the lynched person. They rationalize their actions as being of social value, saying that they wish to deter others, to hasten the slow steps of justice, etc.

It will therefore be of the most vital importance for teachers in the schools of the future to have a means of interpreting any peculiarities of behaviour on the part of the pupil, to the end that they may take measures to prevent the further development of that trend of the unconscious which is indicated by the observed peculiarity. As sadism, or the unconscious desire to inflict cruelty, is a perfectly natural and necessary element in the constitution of the child, but in normal development is outgrown, any person giving evidence by his conscious words or acts of such an unconscious desire is but manifesting the fact that, in this respect, his development has been arrested.

Accordingly it is extremely important, if education is to do the best for the pupil, for some steps to be taken to remove this unconscious desire or to develop it into one of the numerous forms which sublimated sadism takes, such as mastery, leadership, interest in medicine, surgery, etc. In his professional practice, many a surgeon has given a sublimation to the sadistic trend which otherwise would have led him to take pleasure in inflicting pain on other persons and thereby has attained a socially valuable gratification of the unconscious wish.

The teachers of the future will be able to observe and control for the advantage of society this and other trends which give evidence of an irregularity in development.

Thus we see one of the apparent inconsistencies of humans clearly accounted for. The person with an intense, because not seasonably outgrown *desire,* which is yet unconscious, to *inflict* cruelty on man or animals, gets a reputation for an equally intense *aversion* to cruelty, to which, up to the present time, society has given its approval. It is quite evident here that consciousness and the unconscious are working together, but in an inconsistent manner. The unconscious desires cruelty, but is satisfied with the contemplation of cruelty and the effects of cruelty in and on other persons. It is quite evident, also, where the displacement comes in, and that it is the displacement which enables the conscious and the unconscious mental activities to get on the same track. Cruelty is what the mind is craving. In the case of the openly cruel man who becomes a criminal there occurs too, and without displacement, a uniting of consciousness and the unconscious in one direction, thus avoiding a conflict, but it is a direction inimical to society and society checks it in what manner it can—at present by jailing or killing the cruel one. In the case of the person who is unconsciously craving to inflict cruelty, there is a displacement. The mind feasts on cruelty, but, in order to gain the approval of consciousness, and of society, so that it can go ahead full speed, it displaces the infliction of cruelty from self to some other person, In the case of some surgeons the displacement is of another character, for instead of the unconscious satisfaction being derived from the cruelty itself, the satisfaction is displaced (though not misplaced) to a satisfaction derived from the good results of the actions which cause pain.

This is the displacement of the teacher inflicting corporal punishment. The fancied good result of it replaces in his consciousness the unconscious gratification of his unconscious desire to inflict pain. Because there is supposed to be a good result, the goodness covers in his mind the badness of the cruelty and contributes to the severity of the punishment. This applies of course to all sorts of punishment, and indeed is the fundamental objection against punishment of any kind, whether in school or out. The justice of the retribution covers the desire to inflict pain and reinforces it, and the mind continues to be directed toward the offence, which in many ways would better be ignored entirely.

Like the significance of the occurrence of ideas (page 197), the significance of the mind's being unduly occupied with certain ideas or feelings is very great. In the sadistic persons above mentioned the idea of cruelty or inflicting pain or punishment has seized and has, temporarily at any rate, full possession of the minds of the individuals in question. The very fact that a misdemeanour has been observed by a teacher is sometimes a proof that the teacher has been unconsciously on the lookout for a chance to express his unconscious sadism; and the entire episode of detecting, and of recording and of administering punishment (beautiful phrase!) is an instance of a mild obsession of an idea. The ideas that should be exchanged by teacher and pupil are English, arithmetic, etc., *and* progress—social service. None of these enters into the misdemeanour drama, which is therefore just so much lost time, and worse, for emphasis is thrown on the destructive instead of on the constructive element in the social relation existing between teacher and pupil.

Sublimation

I have several times had occasion to speak of sublimation, which is a kind of displacement. When the surgeon displaces the gratification derived from inflcting pain onto that derived from the results of the inflicting of the pain, which are of advantage to society, he is sublimating a trend of the unconscious. This trend, if left unsublimated and allowed to come directly into consciousness as it does in the murderer, let us say, is opposed to society and renders him an outcast. The thoughts which precede the crime also segregate him from true relations with society even before the crime is committed.

Sadism is only one of the many infantile traits which are manifested not only in but out of school, not only by children but by adults. Another very prominent trait is called " exhibitionism," or the desire to show off. In the actual infant it is evinced in a delight in taking off clothes and running around naked. In adults this also occurs and in some morbid cases constitutes a crime. These are the two extremes of the impulse, both in an unsublimated form. These impulses of sadism and exhibitionism are what are called partial impulses. They might better be called paired impulses. Each one of them occurs always paired with the so-called ambivalent trend. For example, the impulse to exhibit one's person is the ambivalent form of the impulse to look at the persons of others. This tendency to peep has been given legendary expression in the character of the Peeping Tom in the story of Godiva. In that legend the attitude of society toward the adult who retains this infantile trait is expressed by the statement that he was struck blind. For looking at Diana in the bath, Actæon, in Greek myth, was killed by the goddess' dogs.

But the ambivalence is evident. The desire to look presupposes a correlative desire to be looked at. The desire to take pleasure from inflicting pain on others presupposes a correlate in the desire to derive pleasure from having pain inflicted on oneself. So that here we have two infantile psychic trends, both duplex (ambivalent) in nature, and giving, when unequally outgrown, four broad classifications of undeveloped human character. The child who grows up without losing its desire to exhibit itself naked is seen in the woman who takes pleasure (unconscious though it may be) in the wearing of abbreviated attire. It may be said to be a general fact that women are more likely to show this trait than men, as is seen by the difference in the conventional clothing of men and women.

So that the impulse to be seen, viewed in its passive aspect, may be counted as the feminine form of this pair of impulses, both of which are, however, in every human psyche, even in adults, more or less sublimated. And the impulse to see, as an active trend, is correspondingly a masculine trait, sublimated more or less in all humans, whether men or women. It should never be forgotten that before the age of puberty the characteristics of boys and girls are predominantly active and passive, but cannot be called really masculine and feminine traits. These traits are not fully developed in the individual until after making the choice of a love object. So that if we remember that these traits are partial trends or ambivalent or paired as I have called them, and that both are in their double or ambivalent form in both sexes, we shall have a clearer idea of the fourfold nature of humanity, any one petal of which, so to speak, may grow to an enlarged condition in either man or woman or all four be discarded or sublimated as they should be in the normally developed adult. In these they are outgrown or discarded if the individual grows up to be an average normal conventional man or woman with no striking peculiarities and doing his work without the desire for more than the usual applause and reward.

If, on the other hand, a person is distinguished for his desire to appear in public, then his exhibitionistic trait has been more or less sublimated or made socially available according to the real value placed on it by society, a value which sometimes cannot be immediately estimated. A great actor is an example of a successful sublimation of the exhibitionistic trend. But it is nevertheless the sublimation of an infantile trait which is possessed by the average adult only in rudimentary form, like the appendix vermiformis. The sublimation *is* the employment by society. Society therein selects certain individuals whom, so to speak, it licenses, by paying them good salaries, to retain that particular infantile trait, for its amusement and recreation. Not only does society sublimate or raise up this trait in the great actor, but it may be equally well said, from the point of view of the actor himself, that he sublimates his own early tendency by employing it in a way which will give pleasure and profit to his fellow-men, as indeed it would not, if it were not transmuted, by this subliming process, by being constantly directed with unremitting effort to the requirements of the social environment. Thus we may either say that the actor is lifted by society or that he raises himself by adapting his desires to the desires of society in such a way that he can continue to get pleasure from a source whence the average man has long since ceased to derive it—from being looked at. But whether the actor lifts himself or is lifted by society, the infantile desire is said to be sublimated.

Just as in the case of the sadist, or person occupied with cruelty, the anti-vivisectionist activities are displacement, so, in the case of exhibitionism, the histrionic activities are a displacement. The pleasure which the unsublimated desire would find in merely being looked at is reinforced by the idea that some other end than merely being looked at is being attained at the same time. The approval of society shown in its being willing to look and be entertained is a cover for the pleasure itself and under this cover the individual seems to get society's orders to go ahead full speed with the acting and the unconscious of the actor achieves the gratification of its desire.

There is a difference in degree, however, between the sadist sublimated slightly to an anti-vivisectionist or to an inventor of improved methods for executing criminals and the sadist who is sublimated greatly into a very successful surgeon. Society does not grant the anti-vivisectionist a very great reward, either spiritual or material, for his degree of sublimation, while to the surgeon it gives a very substantial recognition both in money and fame. I might go on and show that the exact parallel between sublimation and social approval is so exact that the sublimation of a trend of the psyche is nothing more or less than the selection by society of that particular trend for its own use or amusement. This shows very clearly the relation of society, not to the individual as a whole but to certain elements in his character; that is, society's relation to parts of individuals. For its own purposes society takes these traits in different individuals and develops them or transmutes them into their sublimations.

Another illustration of the sublimation of the exhibition impulse is found in pictorial art. The sculptor, painter or draughtsman has transmuted his desire to be seen into a desire to have the work of his hands seen. By the analogical reasoning the work of the artist is in a certain sense himself. There lies the displacement in this case. The work takes the place of the worker. In his thought the worker is displaced by his work. In the work he can get a full gratification of his craving to be seen, a desire which is reinforced by the approbation which he may win from the public. His craving to be seen is uplifted by society from the crass infantile exposition of his naked body in which he delighted when three or four years old to the sublimated form of exhibiting in a certain sense his naked soul, a sublimated form of exhibition because society, of which he is a part, has picked out this trait and marked it as useful for its purposes.

The point of this lengthy analysis of the partial or

ambivalent impulses, one member of each pair being always in the unconscious, is that in one sense a real education is exactly this same sublimation of the natural instincts or, as will immediately be seen, the socialization of the natural instincts. Without this aim education is indeed a misnomer, for it does not draw out and develop innate desires, adapting them to its special needs, but superimposes a foreign body like a veneer. So that we now have something to add to the original definition of education with which we started. We began by saying that the purpose of education was to transform physical energy into mental energy, and we now see that to do it properly it has not only to be transformed but also to be adapted, that is, transformed according to a pattern which is made for it by society, or in other words sublimated. So that the aim of education is the sublimation or adaptive transformation of physical into psychical energy.

It is not necessary to suppose that a complete sublimation of *all* the unconscious craving for life, love and activity can be or need be made in the case of each individual. Only the surplus energy, which is indeed very great, is necessary to be sublimated. H. G. Wells in several of his books remarks upon the fact that much of the misery in the world comes from the surplus vitality of mankind and says that the great problem is to turn it from destructive to constructive lines.

It will be seen that this sublimation does not necessarily always imply the transformation of the physical to the mental energy. Purely physical energy can be sublimated without turning it into mental energy. The physical work of the digger of ditches, which is presumably the extreme type of socialized physical energy, is a sublimation in that it serves society, while if a man of equal physique spaded sand all day long on the sea-shore for the waves to wash smooth again, he would not be sublimating because his actions would not be related to society's needs.

Thus sublimation is seen to lift an individual up out of the narrow limitations of his otherwise isolated self, and unite him with his fellows on a plane higher than that on which he would be living in solitariness. The digger of ditches does, to be sure, a certain small amount of mental work in digging along a line, but here the physical is so great in proportion to the mental that the latter can almost be ignored. It cannot be abso-lutely ignored, however, because it is only the fact that he is following the line that constitutes the social ele-ment of his actions. At the other extreme is the draughtsman in whom the physical energy is all trans-muted, save that portion which holds him in his chair and his hand in the proper position. Both the digger of ditches and the draughtsman are sublimating their ex-cess vitality, the former without and the latter with a transformation of physical into mental energy.

The transition from physical to mental activity can be made in an instant; by man and by animals in the most natural situations it is made in a twinkling, as is illustrated in the change from running to watching. In running we may say that all the energies of the organ-ism are directed outward; and when the animal sud-denly stops in some covert and crouches watching intently to see if his pursuer has followed or missed his trail, we may say that only a small portion of his activities are directed outward, only his vision. His energy is instantaneously converted from purely physical to the nearest to mental this side of truly abstract thinking. Children at play similarly alternate between activity and passivity, in which there is observable a certain degree of 'mental activity.

But the mentality contained in these passive interludes in the rhythm of activity and passivity is very slight and rarely has the quality of directed thinking. Thinking of the directed variety, however, is really a very strenuous activity, so that it is almost the equivalent in actual energy of a fight or a flight of the active kind. This is the kind of mental activity which in school we expect and demand that the pupil carry on. The transition from physical to mental activity of the undirected kind is readily made by all humans alike, young or old. It is taking place daily and hourly out of school. But in school we are looking for the impossible if we expect to see the transition instantaneously made from physical activity to directed mental activity. My idea is that, in the schools of the future, sublimation will be easily and normally effected to very high levels by combining physical activity and directed mental activity in a proportion such that at first the directed mental element will be very slight. The next grade of advance will lessen the former and increase the latter very slightly and so on until the proportions are exactly as desired. I doubt whether this can ever be done in classes at wholesale, because the rate of transition to directed mental activity varies so greatly in individuals.

In an education that has for its problem the transformation from physical to directed mental activity the sublimation of the purely physical has to be neglected. That is what distinguishes the so-called cultural or academic from vocational education, which has for its aim the sublimation of the purely physical activity, and from technical education, which aims at a directed mental activity having for its object the improvement in methods and productiveness of the physical activity.

The great fallacy which has dominated the thinking of all men for so many centuries is that the submission of the purely physical is of a lesser value than that of the purely mental. There is no proof that it is. One might find very good arguments to prove quite the contrary. Man has a physical nature which the purely mental tends to repress, making the body a damaged article through neglect. A proper proportion of the mental and physical makes for a longer, happier and more useful life. But society has for centuries more richly rewarded the mental than the physical worker, indicating that this is the line in which social evolution is progressing. So possibly it is inevitable that a higher value must always be set on directed thinking than on directed doing, though it seems to me that the value really should be different and not higher, for if all eventually should attain this end of sublimated, directed mental activity, the physical medium with which life is carried on would sensibly deteriorate and with it the mentality. The supposition that one kind of activity is better or higher than another is, then, a fallacy. Having a mind inseparably during life connected with a body, we have no right to develop the one at the expense of the other. We shall eventually, then, have to be able to tell a person when he is young whether he belongs in the class which is capable of having his physical energy transformed into mental energy or not. If he is not, we shall have to learn how to persuade him not to try to sublimate the wrong kind of energy. Fortunately a goodly number of young persons realize at some time during their schooling that they can more readily sublimate their physical than their mental activities, and relieve themselves and their teachers of the unpleasant duty of telling them so. But there are many yet remaining in the academic institutions whose time is woefully wasted in fruitless attempt to transform their physical energy into mental energy, an attempt which is worse than fruitless in one sense because the discouragement which they experience in trying to do what is impossible for them diffuses itself over their whole life.

Diffuse Displacement

A form of displacement called diffuse displacement does indeed occur very commonly in normal life and quite as commonly in the schoolroom. It is the tendency to find fault with everything. The cause of it is a defect in the fault-finder. This depends upon the principle (page 158) that it is impossible to see in the external world what does not already exist in the mind. An infant playing on the edge of a parapet over which a fall would be fatal does not see the danger. The ability to see the danger is entirely a matter of mental development. The person long experienced in automobile driving does not " see danger " in this form of locomotion as does one who has never driven in a motor car. He may have seen danger in the days when he was learning to drive, but he has, if not neurotic, developed beyond the seeing of danger in this activity. What he sees, as is well known, is a great many things which his inexperienced passenger could not see in the short time they are visible. He sees, in other words, things he has formerly seen and in a sense never anything absolutely new.

This principle applies with peculiar aptness to one's inability to criticize anything in another person, without having in his own conscious or unconscious mental life the same defect as that criticized. This principle, too, if fully realized by all people, would finally cut out all censorious criticism from the social relations of all people. If we fully believed and clearly saw that we could never find a fault in another which we didn't have in ourselves, we would then keenly appreciate the fact that every time we found fault with anyone we were advertising the existence of that in ourselves too.

While there are doubtless many apparent exceptions to this principle, I think it is undoubtedly true in the broad aspects of human character. The boy who goes around with a chip on his shoulder is generally pretty sure of a fight. Any person who is " looking for trouble " frequently, to say the least, finds it. It illustrates the form of displacement which is technically known as the " projection of a reproach." A person has an unconscious feeling of guilt. Unconsciously he feels that he is a coward. Displacing this feeling (a displacement which occurs in the unconscious) to others, he acts toward them as if they were cowards—acts, in other words, as if he were a bully himself. Thus it is when a bully is really tested by a fearless opponent his essential sense of inferiority is manifested and he runs. The aggressive acts of the bully are really an over-compensation for his unconscious feeling of inferiority. Of course he is unaware of his true inferiority. He sincerely and firmly believes, for the greater part of the time, that he is physically superior. The same thing, too, applies to the intellectual bully. His sense of inferiority is only unconscious. It may then be asked, what is the importance of another person's knowing this, if the physical or mental bully is himself deceived about his own essential inferiority. It certainly will not influence him to be told that he is at heart a coward. He has probably been told that many times already. I offer it, however, as another example of the conscious mind being occupied by or seized by a certain kind of thought like the persons (the sadistic characters mentioned on page 142) whose thoughts are mostly of cruelty. The bully is one who thinks too much about physical prowess. The mechanism is that his essential inferiority, of which he has been of course absolutely unaware, has caused him, though he did not know why, to think about physical superiority. The bully may be made originally in childhood by a beating at the hand of an older and stronger person. From that time on, and particularly if his mind has had no chance of ingesting other ideas on account of the exigencies of his environment, he thinks of personal encounters in which of course he always fancies himself the victor.

Just as the bully will criticize his coevals for their alleged cowardice until they become tired about hearing about such a topic and squelch him, so any person, if he be naïve enough to find fault with any others, will criticize them only for the faults which he has himself. And yet he is not conscious of having those faults himself. The only way he becomes conscious of the faults is when he attributes them to other people. But in attributing them to other people he is, of course, explicitly declaring those faults to be the other people's and not his own. The very necessity of attributing them to other people is an effort to get rid of, to foist upon others, what is really his own. He thus expresses his desire to be free from those defects. That is his way of freeing himself from those faults—by shoving them off onto other people.

Here we see how purely a matter of wishing it is, how the act of criticizing or fault-finding is the conscious expression of the unconscious desire to have the virtues which are the opposites of those vices which are blamed in others. Thus only can we become conscious of our own faults—when we find that we have attributed them to others. So that when Brown says, "Smith is an ill-tempered man," he should add, "which shows that I am ill-tempered in noting it in him." If Owen More says: "Old Gotrox is a detestable miser," he should add, in order to tell the whole truth, "but my remark shows that I am stingy myself, or I should never have thought it of him." If Mrs. McCray Fish says, "That Miss Arma Dillo has a perfectly horrid nature," she must, in order to include all that accusation implies, continue, "but, of course, I suppose I'm a mean thing myself to be saying so."

If we are sufficiently well read in human nature to interpret the manifold displacement mechanisms of the mind, we shall now clearly see that almost all statements *about* human nature involve displacements of one kind or another. And in the sphere of human mental qualities we cannot, without realizing the universality of this mechanism, get the full sense of the statement that almost nothing that a man, woman or child can say about their own or their neighbours' characters, mental or spiritual, can possibly be the truth. In matters of pure human nature nobody naturally tells the truth. They think they want to, but they are completely turned about by their own unconscious wishes. Whatever one says is almost sure to be quite the opposite of the truth. We can tell the concrete facts, such as the time of day or the measures of things, although scientists will there remind us that the constant error and the personal equation are inevitable in all judgments of quality.

In the schoolroom we find the displacements rampant and uncorrected both in teacher and in pupil. The teacher, if disposed to be critical, judges according to the social standard with which she is herself familiar. She notices in pupils only the deportment which she is trained in, qualified to examine and report upon. Of course she sees only the fine qualities she herself has. But having them, there is no unconscious urge to transfer or displace them to others and so praising others is not instinctively strained after by the unconscious. Only the Omnipotent can see that everything is good. The partipotent can see only the fragments of the goodness of the earth or the inhabitants thereof. The beauty is in the eye of the beholder in a very literal sense.

The most deficient classes in school are those whose members are always looking out for unfairness, partiality, dishonesty and misbehaviour on the part of the other members of the class. The displacements are legion. Their minds are more occupied with moral than with intellectual questions, because they are themseleves more immoral than the classes whose minds are more occupied with the subject-matter of their lessons. True occupiedness with their lessons crowds out questions of deportment or dishonesty, and no accusations are made. On the other hand, the teacher that is a martinet in discipline shifts the mental activity from the intellectual to the moral question, much to the detriment of the school work. True work truly accomplished is honesty itself.

If the relations between teacher and pupil *could* be intellectual relations only, if the minds of both parties *could* be entirely occupied with the subject-matter of the course of study during the time supposed to be devoted to it, the displacements would be avoided. These displacements are, however, universal unconscious mental mechanisms, and themselves partly constitute the real cause why an absolutely unified relation cannot exist between the pupil and the work. There are many other determinants, one of which is mentioned (page 194) as the unconscious wish to do something of real present value, and the knowledge, partly conscious but progressively more and more repressed, that the activities of the school work are of no real present value. If ever they ask what is the *use* of studying this and that, the children are told that it trains their minds and that a well-trained mind will be at some time in the future a great advantage to them, and they will be much better able to gain at that future time what they will want at that future time. But, to the unconscious, present wants alone have dynamic force to cause action. The unconscious is unoriented toward time or reality. It knows no future, and it only wishes, and in terms of the present.,

So that from one point of view we are in present education attempting to substitute a future want for a present want, a sort of displacement designed to drive out the other natural and unconscious displacements so characteristic of all human undirected thinking or phantasying (wishing expressed in mental images). This may be considered analogous to the self-denial which, according to the principles of political economy, we suppose to be necessary for a man to exercise in order to create capital. He denies himself a present small gratification, saving a penny now in order to have a pound later.

This is a very difficult thing to do, because it is absolutely contrary to the trends of the unconscious wish, which always presses for present gratification. As we have seen, one of the commonest forms of displacement is an unconscious replacement of one idea containing the external form of a wish by another idea which is somewhat similar to it. The form of the original wish, for instance the desire to be cruel, is contrary to the requirements of society, while the substituted wish form, for instance the desire to perform surgical operations, is in conformation with the requirements of society.

The displacement is the acceptance of the one wish for the other and the ignorance that in the second wish form the original wish is to a certain extent satisfied. It is much as if the person had a strong desire to push or to pull, and that desire could be turned to good advantage by getting him to push a hand-cart or to pull a wagon. The unconscious, while always in a state exactly analogous to a supposed person wanting merely to pull and not wanting to pull any particular thing, is never unaccompanied by consciousness in some form, which always gives a definite shape to the desire to pull. The wish has a form given to it by the physical constitution of the individual who is the stage whereon the wishes appear. If an individual is endowed with a strong physique, he will desire to use it, to use all his muscles and send things flying. If he has a big voice, he will want to use it; if he has an eye sensitive to shades of colour, he will want to work in colour in some way. Also his mental experiences will give form to his wishes, as we very familiarly see when a child has a new experience and wishes immediately to repeat it. If by his parents this new experience is considered good, i.e. advantageous to society as they understand it, the wish to repeat it will be gratified; but if considered disadvantageous, an immediate substitution or displacement is consciously made by the parents. A baby wants to suck its thumb, and either a pacifier is given to it, or a pair of spherical metal gauntlets is put on its hands. The pacifier satisfies its desire to suck and saves the thumb from being deformed but not the mouth. The gauntlets are interesting in quite another manner, and so satisfy a craving, but not the original one. The form of the first craving is displaced by that of the second, though in a sense it may be said that the craving is essentially the same in either case. The indirection is a mark of the substitution. The baby does not know or does not appear to know the difference.

We are all in the baby's position in all of the unconscious substitutes made for our gratification by society and environment. We do not know the difference. We are satisfying our primordial craving every moment * (yes, even in vehemently expressing our dissatisfaction), though we do not know that it is the unconscious wish that we are satisfying and not the conscious desire which alone we think we are satisfying.

Exactly the same thing is going on in every schoolroom every minute. Not only the unconscious displacements, about which the pupil knows nothing and which are supplied by the environment, but the consciously intended displacements which the teacher is constantly endeavouring to make, and which are unconsciously resisted by the pupil.

Rationalization

A man who smoked more tobacco than he thought he ought to began to cut down on his cigars on account of expense. He preferred cigars to tobacco in any other form, but smoked a pipe for economy, getting, however, a certain amount of real pleasure from it. Though still longing for cigars, which he used to buy by the box, and of the ten-cent quality, he persistently, after his resolution, refrained from buying a box of them, knowing that he would smoke six a day, a waste of money which he could ill afford. He would buy two ten-cent cigars on his way home and smoke one after dinner, keeping the next for next day's dinner. Then he would see this cigar after breakfast the next morning, and would smoke it. Thereafter he would buy only one ten-cent

* I shall have a great deal more to say about the continual satisfaction of unconscious wishes on pages 167 and 257.

cigar. Later he felt so virtuous about this economy that he thought if he denied himself two cigars a day he might as well have a moderately good one (this was before the war), and would buy a fifteen-cent cigar. Occasionally thereafter he would omit a day for some reason, either that he did not happen to pass the usual cigar store or that he was in a hurry and did not want to take time.

Once he was met at the train by his daughter, who walked home with him. They had an errand on the opposite side of the street from the cigar store. As they started to cross, she said to him: " Aren't you going to get your cigar? " He took this as an excuse, as he did everything that came along and bought one at another store they passed, but compromised with himself and bought a ten-cent cigar instead of a fifteen-cent one. The next day when he was trying to pass the cigar store the thought came to him: " You had only a poor cigar last night. You might get a fifteen-cent one now, to make up for it."

He had occasional headaches which his conscience suggested to him came from too much smoking. But he also had a slight indigestion now and then, and his desire for cigars suggested that the headaches might just as well come from the indigestion and have nothing to do with tobacco, and so then he would buy and smoke a cigar. It then came into his mind that if there was any doubt about it, he could prove it by quitting smoking for a time, and see if he had any headaches. The idea that the tobacco might also cause the indigestion never occurred to him.

Finally he became disgusted with the reasons which he

was habitually giving to himself for smoking, and saw
that any reason whatever was reason enough to induce
him to smoke, and that as a matter of fact one reason
was just as good as another. His reasons in other
words were really as rational as those giving excuses
to the drinker for imbibing, in the following old dog-
gerel:

> *If all be true that I do think,*
> *There are five reasons we should drink:*
> *Good wine, a friend, or being dry,*
> *Or lest we may be by and by,*
> *Or any other reason why.*

The motive force of the reason is therefore dependent
not on the reason itself, but on the desire to drink, or,
in the case of the man above referred to, the desire to
smoke cigars. In other words, the so-called reason,
which should in reality be a cogent reason, or one compelling the man to do something, was in this case merely
the act that released a great force of desire into external
realization. Any fact, whether relevant or not, was
used as an excuse. " Any other reason why " would do
as well as the legitimate reason for smoking a cigar, if
there *was* any legitimate reason.

One might safely make a general statement that anything will satisfy us as a reason to justify us in doing anything we want to do. There are two factors in this
situation, both of which should be mentioned: first that
there is no difference in the quality of reasons accepted
by people for doing what they want to do, and second
that they universally feel this need of justifying an action
which at the same time they feel to be unwise. We are

all giving ourselves or other people reasons which we offer in defence of our actions (and of course we think some at least of them need defence) because we feel that we need to give reasons for our actions. This practically universal tendency to justify our actions, or our thoughts on verbal principles, is known as *rationalization*.

The rationalizations of the cigar smoker above mentioned were conscious ones. He knew that in a sense he was fooling himself all the time. But the majority of rationalizations are, in the case of most people, entirely unconscious. People do not know that the reasons they give for a statement or an opinion or an action are dictated to them by their own unconscious, and that their apparent cogency is attributable solely to their congruence with the desires of the people giving them as reasons. If we realize the fact that most reasons are mere rationalizations, we shall soon clearly see that in nine cases out of ten the reasons assigned by persons for doing anything are not the real causes why they do those things, but are indirect expressions of the unconscious wish. It is quite enlightening to realize that if you are unacquainted with your own unconscious, not a single reason you can possibly assign for anything you think, say or do is the *real cause* of your thinking, saying or doing it. The real cause is the unconscious wish of which you cannot possibly, without a thorough study of your own unconscious, be aware in the least degree. Only after a thorough analysis by an expert analyst can you trace any of your actions to their true cause.

This gives a clear exposé of the absolute futility of asking a child why he did such and such a thing—for instance, committed some form of disorder. He does not know and could not tell if he tried. Some will simply sit or stand mute, looking on the floor. Others will fabricate more or less glib excuses which are, to the teacher, quite manifestly mere excuses, while those who are less sophisticated will feel miserable because they think the teacher wants them to say something and they cannot do so. Why they did not study their lessons, why they made this or that mistake, etc., all are quite as much unknown to them as are the real causes of his action to the habitual rationalizer.

From this human tendency to rationalize every one of their acts emerges the fact that all people do what they want to and subsequently seek to align their actions with the principles of social living by assigning reasons for doing what they want to do.

And from this it appears that whatever people are doing is what they want to do. This is the fact which is hardest to believe of all the facts recently discovered about the human soul. If it is true that all wishes are gratified in one of two ways, either consciously or unconsciously (page 257), it is also true that whatever people are doing all the time is fulfilling their wishes. It seems quite an outrage on common sense to suppose that a poor man is poor because he wants to be poor, or that a sick man is sick because he wants to be sick, or that an unfortunate wants to be unfortunate; but it is the literal truth. Only we must remember that in being poor, sick or unfortunate it is frequently only the unconscious wish that is being fulfilled, and there are different degrees of unconsciousness in wishes.

If the particular man is utterly unaware of any possible advantage that could come to him from his being sick, his wish which is being fulfilled is totally unconscious. If the particular person who is poor cannot possibly imagine any advantages in being poor, his wish to be poor is only an unconscious one. But there are many poor men who have found compensations or who have said that they found compensations in poverty; and, as for the unfortunate, why, " Sweet are the uses of adversity," words from a speech which is a beautiful example of rationalization, for in that soliloquy the duke is merely justifying his own inactivity and his submissiveness to the stronger will of his brother.

It has been proved that many accidents resulting in injury have been in reality merely the fulfilment of unconscious wishes of the person injured, if he was the cause of the accident, or of the causer of the accident, if the person who was injured was in any way inimical to him. The fact is recognized in law in the term " criminal negligence." It might almost be said that every catastrophe except some cases of death by lightning is the expression of some unconscious wish of some person or group of persons. I groan under the present conditions of the high cost of living, and I know full well that I am not doing a thing to prevent it, and that I must wish it, at any rate unconsciously, more than a low cost, or at any rate I and all the others who similarly groan are desiring other things which we devote our energies to getting, more than we would the getting of the low cost, or we would all unite and get it.

The axiom that what we are getting is the actual fulfilment of our conscious or unconscious wishes is of extreme interest in that other but immured little world of the schoolroom.

What the pupils are doing is what they wish to do in spite of all external control, suggestive or dogmatic. And at the same time they are being trained in rationalization. Those who are naïve enough to give expression to every wish which emerges into their consciousness are at once reprimanded and the unconscious wish, instead of becoming conscious in its original form, is displaced to some other form. Its unconscious nature is concealed and its unconscious form is no longer known. The unconscious wishes are banned as unspeakable, horrible. They must be put out of sight. They must be put in a place where we cannot know about them any longer, not even what they do to us without our knowledge. That attitude is about as sensible as turning our backs on a wild beast in a forest, so that we could put him out of sight and out of mind.

Pupils in schools are trained in rationalization, for they are permitted to do what they wish, and no power can prevent them, and they are questioned and reasoned with and taught to give the wrong reasons for their acts. An unconscious wish can be fulfilled by an act which is composite in its nature, partly conscious and partly unconscious, the conscious element of it representing the compliance with the school situation and the unconscious element being there all the time and constituting the fulfilment of the unconscious wish. Thus a boy may be told to leave the room, and he leaves it, complying with the request, and apparently not fulfilling any unconscious wish, because he is being disgraced and placed in a situation of inferiority. But he makes faces and walks slowly to the door and slams it when he goes out, thus fulfilling his conscious desire to get even with the teacher, and his unconscious desire to exhibit.

In a state of society there are no simple acts. All are composite. If there were only two people in the world, and they lived within each other's perception, nothing that one of them did would be without its effect on himself and on the other. In a schoolroom of forty pupils there may be 1,600 motives for a child's doing one thing or another, if by motive we imply causes both in the child and in the environment.

When I said that what the pupils are doing is what they wish to do, I mean of course what they unconsciously wish to do. Consciously they may very keenly wish to do something other than what they are doing, but in the condition of being baffled in their conscious wishes not to go to school, or not to learn that particular lesson, or even in their conscious wish to excel in the subject they are still studying, they are in a condition where the unconscious wishes are much more likely to be expressed (in a disguised form, of course). When anyone is baffled, all the inceptive movements, which in the successful activity here obstructed are necessarily retained within the organism, struggle to issue into the external world in forms, popularly described as fidgeting, fussing or uneasy motions, forms of motion which are nothing but a more direct expression of the unconscious wish than would be the case if the attempted action which is being obstructed had not been begun. In a sense fidgeting is a more unconscious action than a great many others. We do not foresee each motion as we do when we are doing something according to a plan, and we sometimes do not know what we are doing at the very time when we are doing it. When we are doing something according to a plan we have an additional means of remembering it other than ordinary retentiveness; and after fidgeting awhile we can rarely remember what we have done. Thus the uneasiness of children in a schoolroom is a direct manifestation of the unconscious wish.

Summary

In this chapter we have seen that *identification*, a fundamental mechanism based on similarity, is further differentiated into *projection* and *introjection*, and that both of these are entirely unconscious; we have seen that *compensation* is a conscious tendency balancing an unconscious one, that this compensation is mediated through the *displacement* of ideas, and that *rationalization* is an ingrained habit of humanity to give, after an action, a reason for it which is never the true cause of the action. To the concept of *libido* as a creative wish is added the consideration that it may be *sublimated* or devoted to aims essentially non-sexual but productive. All these mechanisms are as clearly in evidence in the schoolroom as anywhere else, and it is a very great advantage for the teacher to become aware of them.

CHAPTER VI

THE AIM OF EDUCATION

AFTER twenty years of teaching in a secondary school I am convinced that the modes of thinking on the part of many children are irremediably (without the teacher's knowing of the effects of the unconscious) twisted, and that they are so by virtue of their numerous complexes. I have seen class after class of bright-looking children, both girls and boys, develop utterly unnecessary and retarding resistances against not only my own but other subjects. Repeatedly in the classroom I have developed the fact that the pupils perfectly well knew what was necessary in order to express themselves tersely and clearly. But I have found that the pupils are governed by an unconscious wish *not* to make a good showing in school, *not* to perform thoroughly and well the tasks set. There exists a deep-rooted unconscious desire to undervalue the academic training and to exaggerate its difficulties, partly, no doubt, because of the parental point of view that the curriculum is too long or too complicated, and partly because of the unconscious resistance to authority of any kind—a resistance which is natural to all humans.

But the main point to be emphasized in this chapter is the fact of the very early determination of these traits by the ill-advised (or, better, un-advised) actions of parents. Much has been written about the unfortunate results of neglecting adenoids, enlarged tonsils, defective teeth and eyes, but very little upon the purely mental aspect of the problem.

Early Impressions

And first of all it is not generally understood, either by parents or teachers, how supremely important are the impressions received by the boy or girl at the very inception of mentality, that is, during the first years of life —from one to five years of age.

The period of the child's life before it is old enough even to go to kindergarten is in all ways the most important in its life in the dominating effect it has on the major traits of character of later years. The child is impressed by everything, and particularly by the moods and manners of the personal environment, impressed in ways and to a degree hitherto unrecognized, impressed so forcibly that on the plastic material, through which the soul is expressed, an almost permanent matrix is imprinted the changes in which wrought by subsequent events are of well-nigh negligible value.

The design of that matrix consists largely of affective material, or is really an affective pattern. It is as if the temperament was fixed at that early age, the tendency to be extraverted or introverted finally determined, the respect for authority created (or ever after lost), and in general the social or asocial nature of the individual's reactions to his human environment are moulded in the pre-school days in such a way that they automatically colour and modify all the individual's later acts.

If the child has both parents who are sexually well

mated, there results in the home atmosphere so invigorating an air of satisfaction and comfort and love that the child's own nature is inspired into being warm and sunny. If, on the other hand, the child has for parents a married couple between whom there is not a complete physical and spiritual union, there is lacking for his own subsequent love-life an important, indeed essential, element, a lack which is perceived by the child at once, whether consciously or unconsciously. In this case the child lacks at least a part of one parent, is, let us say, three-quarters parented (to make a verb out of a noun), or three-eighths parented.

Now, the pattern for the subsequent love-life of the boy or girl is imprinted upon his soul by the unconscious perceptions of the child before the age of five, possibly three, and whether he sleeps in the same room with his parents or not, he will unconsciously perceive and unconsciously interpret the symbolism of the actions of his parents in relation to each other. He will perceive how and in what tone of voice they address each other, and will know, unconsciously to be sure, whether there is in that tone the full sonority of the persons whose love is entirely and completely devoted to the love of the soul as well as body mate. Even if these perceptions are unconscious for years or forever, they will determine the adolescent's attitude toward persons of the opposite sex.

Confidence

For it is in these earliest years that sexual confidence is developed or stunted, and it is accelerated or retarded solely by observation of the sexual confidence on the part

of those by whom the child's earliest years are influenced.
To take only one instance, the habit of looking squarely
into the eyes of another is a sign of the greatest love
significance. The eye is, above all other features of
the face, the truest indication of love power. The eye
that shifts *from* the gaze of another is the gaze of a child
who, by the parents or their surrogates in its earliest
years, has been shamed, punished, ridiculed, shocked or
what not. The eye, on the other hand, which shifts
toward the eye of another is the eye of a child which
has been brought up in confidence, and has not met the
blasting rebuffs which destroy the unity of love by taking
from it one of its truest outlets.

Thus one might characterize even adults as being the
possessors of the approaching glance or the fleeing
glance. The person with the coming eye looks frequently *into* the eyes of his companion. He does not
look, as some do hastily, *at* them and as hastily avert
his gaze. Nor of course does he stare, an act whose
symbolism is quite different at different stages of spiritual
development. The " baby stare " is an opening of, and
direction of, the eyes largely for the purpose of being
looked at. It has been recorded of a modern pugilist
that his eyes by their fierceness frequently helped to quell
his adversaries, and Caesar, in telling of the mutiny
which almost occurred in his army when it was approaching the soldiers of Ariovistus, mentions the fact that his
own men were disconcerted by the tales of the traders,
who said that there were few who could stand up against
the keen glance of the savages' eyes.

In what way the child that is imperfectly parented will
later register in his own love-life the rate or degree of

his parentedness has been very clearly shown by numerous researches into the unconscious mentality of *only* children or *favourite* children.

Influence of Parents

To the pre-adolescent boy the father or father surrogate becomes the model of what all fathers should be and indeed *are* in the wish-content of his own unconcious, and upon his father's attitude toward the boy's mother depends largely his own later attitude toward his own wife. The fact that parents think their children do not observe and mentally comment upon their parents' actions leads the parents only too late to control themselves in the presence of their children. Thus if there is any reason why the parents should repress any feeling they have for each other, such as momentary irritation or chronic hatred, they will not do so before an infant, and only begin to suspect an influence on the child when he begins to make remarks about the parents' actions or is noticeably troubled by them.

To the pre-adolescent boy, again, the mother or mother surrogate is a model of all a mother should be, and is the indelible prototype of what he is unconsciously looking for in a woman when later he desires a mate of his own. Indeed, it may be said that the idea of taking a mate is not unconsciously (though it may be consciously by his friends, when it naturally meets with the resistance of the unwarmed unconscious) suggested to the young person *until* he or she meets the mother or father replica. It is to be remembered that the mother impression on the unconscious is that of a *young* woman and not a woman of the age of the mother at the time when the youth is inspired to take a wife.

It is this indelible, though unconscious, prototype, still existing in the bottom of his heart, which causes him to be attracted by some girls more than by others. If he finds a girl whose qualities perfectly fit this unconscious maternal matrix, which is forming all his preferences, he falls completely in love with her, and gives expression to this desire in ways which characterize the other mechanisms of his psychic-physical organism.

This is but another way of saying a boy's first love is his mother. It might be inferred from this that a boy's only love is his mother, but this would be true only in the sense that he loves his wife as he did his mother, or for the same qualities that he perceived in his mother. Here it should be noted, too, that this manner of sex gratification has nothing detrimental about it, unless, as is frequently the case, it involves the *rejection* of other qualities. Then the predominance of this maternal image is truly a misfortune.

Similarly a girl's first love is her father. For to the pre-adolescent girl, not only is her mother the model of all that a mother should be (for whence is she to derive any other models?) but her father is the ideal of all that a father should be (at the early age of one to five what other can she have?) and all her father's actions are unconsciously noted and recorded by her. And how can it be otherwise? Have we not later, even in adulthood, understood the significance of what we have seen earlier, and even forgotten? Does not the significance of a present fact depend upon and come, if not wholly, at least partly, from the unconscious content of the mind which perceives the fact? Therefore to the girl baby whose father whines or scolds at her mother, that type of action, if repeated at any later time by her husband, will arouse in her the same resentment which she felt, and felt her mother feel, when she was a baby.

If she had a father who was cheerful and unruffled, and later finds in her husband a temper uncheerful and irritable, she will not feel toward him the same resentment, because resentment is not a part of her nature. It was not aroused in her infancy by the resentment of a woman expressed against an unreasonable man. In the place of resentment there may occur surprise and an immediate determination to learn and remove the cause, neither of which would occur to the adult trained as a child in the expressions of ill-feeling. The one child is by its environment habituated at the age of one to five years to respond to a situation in a complaining or destructive way. To the other child that way does not occur, but only the constructive way.

And if, furthermore, her father was in her infancy a jolly, unruffled, positive, creative man, she will not regard as men others who have not some approach to these qualities. Unless they strike that chord of robust and cheerful manliness which was strung and struck in the days when she first began to see and hear, she will not notice the man as being worthy of her attention.

As for the young woman, so for the young man, the very quality which makes a member of the other sex stand out as being different from other men and women, making other men and women all alike, is that quality or group of qualities which distinguished the father or mother and made them so exceedingly superior to other persons in the infancy of the young woman or man in question.

And just as the girl's mother is her norm of motherhood, she will expect to behave to her own husband and to her own children, not only consciously expect and plan, but unconsciously will behave in such a way that the mode of *her* own behaviour is consistently and completely determined by the mode which has been stamped on her infant soul by the silent, unnoted and unremembered, though none the less potent, observation.

All this has been mentioned with the purpose of trying to make parents and educators realize in a concrete way the plasticity, the consummate retentiveness and the essential permanence of the infant mentality. At its most plastic age it takes the fortuitous impressions of its environment, takes them very deeply and retains them only slightly altered. If the mind of the child were inanimate plaster, it would do the same thing, but being animate plasma it does it more effectively.

So the old maxim, *Maxima* PUERIS *reverentia debetur,* is to be extended to include children of the youngest age. For the parent it may seem almost ludicrous that he or she, with all their weaknesses, is to be regarded as occupying with respect to the child the position of a god, who having not merely procreated its body must now for at least five years keep up a continuous creation of its mind and soul. It is ludicrous if not appalling that so much power for good or ill is placed in the hands and in the very manners, actions, voice, eye glance and hand habit of the parents and immediate human surroundings of the child. In fine, there is absolutely no circumstance from birth until five or six years of

age which can take place within the mental purview
of the child which may not have the effect of turning him
or her in a direction much desired or equally undesired
by the parents.

But lest it may appear to some parents that their conduct, in the presence of the child whose soul they are
engaged in training after having evoked its body, must
be punctiliously *regulated* according to any given set of
rules, it should be emphasized that any kind of conduct,
even if it be rough, is wholesome enough if it be animated
by the proper feelings of love on the part of the parents
and other members of the family—love not merely for
one person but for as many as possible.   Love will dic-
tate the natural and wholesome response to the various
situations.

It is the more evident that the love of the parents for
each other holds a determining power over the destiny
of their children when the more modern psychology
informs us that, if perfectly mated, a couple have no
fears, phobias nor anxieties of a disease-producing kind,
and when we reflect that a nervous constitution on the
part of one or both parents, showing itself in fears or
anxieties, will have the deleterious effect of giving, so
to speak, a timorous or phobic form to the child's mind.
A fear of thunderstorms, observed in a child of a woman
also afraid of celestial pyrotechnics, is sometimes popularly explained on the ground of its being "inherited."
Much that is inherited by children is inherited not
by heredity but through environment.   If we inherit
money, it is from a *testator* who is *deceased.*   If we
inherit traits of character, it may be from those of our
ancestors who are *alive* as well, but truly inherited traits

in this sense will be inherited by us before we are born and not after. On the other hand, the traits which, by a figure of speech, we may call inherited from our parents *after* we are born are the most constructive or destructive inheritances which the child can have.

And it should be recalled by all parents that the actual nervous constitution, which is determined for the child before the hour of birth, is the inheritance of an infinite number of ancestors, all of whom contribute an approximately equal part. No praise or blame can be attached to the parents for any mental trait the child is possessed of at birth. His body and his nervous constitution are the inevitable effect of causes operating from the beginning of evolution.* But the child's body having been delivered, a responsibility at once rests upon the parents of producing, as far as in them lies, a wholesome mental spiritual environment which is to create the mind of the child.

Creation of Mind

The mind of the newborn infant is less in evidence than that of the day-old chick. It seems as if nature, in the case of humans, had intended to use, as a means of producing in them a conscious rational mentality, a period of utter helplessness, in which the actions upon the outside world should be of absolutely no effect, or of no significant effect, and the human chick, instead of beginning to peck and scratch, should be held by the

---

* Only the most modern of obstetricians introduce into this matter any question of praise or blame, when they advise, for an expectant mother, a diet which is designed to make the unborn smaller than it would have been had the mother's nutritional instincts been followed.

force of its own weight in a position in which it should
be, more than all other animals, assailed by, and practically at the mercy of, outside influences, which may
greatly alter its always variable efficiency.

All young animals except the highest mammalia begin
to shift for themselves comparatively soon. The inactivity and receptivity of the human infant make it more
subject than any other animal to the influence of the
group and less to that of the heredity, i.e. innate constitution. If we should call the innately inherited
qualities " vertical " influences, because they come down
from generation to generation, we might call the influences which are exerted by the environment " horizontal "
influences. Then we should be able to express the whole
matter very well by saying that with the " vertical "
influences the parents have almost nothing at all to
do, but with the " horizontal " influences they not only
have a great deal to do, but they begin to have it as
soon as the child is born, they have to have it, whether
they want it or not, and that their responsibility for
their child's welfare is not only instantaneous but continuous and comprehensive, up to the time when it is no
longer possible or desirable for the parents to be the
sole environment of the child. Then other factors enter,
which do not and ought not to belong to the parents.
Then the child has to begin its relations with the community and the state, in order that its life shall not
remain forever at the narrow calibre of the family.

Too much emphasis cannot be laid upon the good or
evil effect exercised upon the whole subsequent lifetime
of the child by the sunny or the " shady " character of
the love influences with which it is surrounded in the

earliest days. The greatest obstacle to the development of a strong wholesome character is the complex; and the emotion of fear which is the result of a feeling of inferiority is the greatest single factor in forming complexes. The wholesome and sunny temperament so productive of health, happiness and prosperity, which more than anything else annihilates wrong and misfortune, is not the result of a perfectly healthy body alone. It is primarily the result of a point of view, an attitude, a disposition, an early fixed impression for which parents exist and for which they are responsible. Children who are physically perfectly healthy frequently lack this proper attitude towards the world, and sometimes even a crippled or blind child, thanks to loving care, has it.

To the shady nature of the love influences emanating from the parents may be attributed their deleterious influences for the following reasons. The fundamental fear, that which produces a feeling of inferiority always avoided by the unconscious of every man, woman or child, is a sexual fear, a fear either of impotence or sexual inferiority, i.e. unattractiveness. Due to our utterly senseless education, a great many perfectly normal persons know little of sexual norms and fancy they have violated some natural sexual law, and of course fear the consequences of that trespass. As their knowledge is indefinite and inaccurate, they fear an indefinite peril. And as the indefinite always looks big, they exaggerate the supposed effects of their transgression sometimes to the degree of becoming despondent over thinking they have committed the " unpardonable sin."

The sexual relations of most parents are such that

they have been trained to shroud them in the blackest obscurity. Many a man has had his married life ruined by thinking that his mother was so pure that she could not have a passionate love for his father, and that no pure woman like her, as he picked out his wife to be, could be passionately attached to him. Therefore he has thought it out for himself, and quite logically deduced his erroneous conclusions from false premises, namely that, as for passionate love, he had either to give it up entirely or go to prostitutes for it, in whom there can be passion but not love. Many a woman too has been brought up under a training which taught her to believe that to feel any passionate love for any man, even her own husband, was wrong and sinful; therefore she repressed it all and took her husband's advances coldly with the idea that if she responded warmly she would be to him as a prostitute and he would neither admire her nor treat her well, and she would be committing a great sin to love her husband passionately as (she imagines) the prostitutes do. And both parents, having this guilty feeling, he that he should not expect his wife to match him in ardour, and she in the unfortunate misapprehension that only prostitutes can eat the true apple of love, have both suffered alike from their lack of sex education, and they pass this on to their children.

The Child's Sexual Curiosity

The child's first conscious thought about itself is where it comes from. As both parents are ashamed of their marital relations, for no matter how hard the conscious life tries to repress, the unconscious goes on the

plan of " all or nothing," and each parent, when confronted by the sweet innocence of a child just beginning
to think, shrinks from trying to impart any of the
secrets of adult love to an infant who evidently cannot
understand.

Suppose a three-year-old child says, " Mommy, where'd
I come from?" it will take a particularly pure and wholesome mind and one free from fear and ignorance to
reply, in a tone quite as bright and fresh as little Billie's,
" You came out of me, honey." Then imagine the
difficulty on the part of most mothers in carrying on
their end of the following conversation:

B. Where did I come out?
M. A part of me opened and you came out head first.
B. How could I do that 'thout hurtin' you?
M. You didn't. It hurt very much.
B. Does it hurt now?
M. No, not a bit.
B. Gee, I must have made a big hole!
M. No, you were quite small, about as big as Mrs.
Smith's baby over on the Boulevard.
B. How big was I? Show me.
M. You were about so long and so big around, about
the size of sister's doll.
B. How did I ever get in there?
M. You grew in there from as big as the point of a
pin.
B. Mow could I breathe inside of you and eat, 'n'
everthin'?
M. I did it for you.
B. How long was I in there?

M. Nine months; about as long a time as from last Christmas until now.

B. Gee, what a long time! Say, Mommy, did you put me there or did I just grow like an apple?

M. Everything like an apple or an animal grows from the melting together of two little seed like things called cells. One comes from the father, the other is in the mother. They are exactly alike and equal.

Those who could carry their end of the conversation up to this point generally break down here. But this is as far as, or farther than, the very young child pursues this inquiry. In all probability the last question would not be asked, for it is found that the amount of information given here is completely satisfactory for a long time. The important point is, however, that the child should be given as much information as he asks for, but no more. In the beginning the child has the utmost confidence in the parents, from whom he receives all physical comforts and necessities. His absolute faith makes him very jealous of anything that looks like a lack of confidence on the part of the parent. He is likely to resent any lack of sincerity on the parents' part in proportion as his confidence in them has been perfect. The least flaw spoils all for him, and particularly in matters which he instinctively feels are most vital to him.

I repeat that the parents' unwillingness frankly to state to their children the truth about their sexual origin is caused by the parents' own shame in feeling that in some way passionate love is sinful and is therefore to be kept concealed from children who can talk. Possibly it is because the parents fear that the children will say

something about it before strangers.   But most likely
it is from a feeling of reluctance to confess before the
so-called innocence of youth what they themselves
erroneously believe to be wrong.

And I repeat also that much harm comes to children
both from the parents' carelessness about their conduct
in the presence of children before they can talk, and their
mendacity after that time.   Unsatisfied sexual curiosity
leads the children, on the other hand, to invent all sorts
of grotesque theories of conception and birth, and to
listen to other children who are variously misinformed.
Many of these birth and conception theories are found
by medical psychologists as nuclei of various phobias
and other forms of neurosis.   The untruthful statements
of parents when they either say they do not know or
repeat the time-worn myth of babies being brought by
the doctor, have the further result of destroying once
and for all the confidence which the child has up to this
time had in the reliability of his parents.   As the destruction of this confidence amounts to the destruction of
every kind of confidence in themselves as well as in every
other person or thing, it is of the utmost importance
for parents so to school themselves that they can keep
their hold upon their children, at least a little beyond the
time of their first sex inquiry.   The child, instead of
being fully parented, is thus in a sense spiritually
orphaned, and at a very early age.

The Effects of Misinformation

The fundamental basis for a wholesome interest in all
things which is the foundation of a sound education in

any line lies in the undoubting knowledge on every child's part as to how, when and where he himself originated. Lacking this he is likely to doubt all things and, not seeing clearly and straight these fundamental facts, he is prone to look at everything with an intellectual strabism.

If a teacher does not receive the child well oriented in these basic truths it is impossible to prevent many children becoming indifferent or perverse in their attitude toward their school work. All the troublesome phenomena of adolescence would be mitigated if the secondary schools could receive children who had been straightened out on matters of sex, but this will be impossible until parents themselves have succeeded in looking at the matter with an " approaching " glance instead of with the " fleeing " one.

Directed vs. Undirected Thinking

The striking difference existing between the atmosphere of a schoolroom where there are pupils of a higher grade and that where lower-grade pupils are confined, is that the older pupils are quieter. They talk less and they move less. The younger the pupils the greater is the instinctive impulse to move some part of the body including the vocal apparatus, all the time. It may be said that the foremost aim of all education is to transmute the young person's primal urge to keep moving physically into a craving to be active mentally. The first is instinctive and the second has to be acquired at great pains. This aim of changing activities from physical, which are natural, to the directed mental activities, which are not natural, implies that it is a desirable aim. Everything that man has done, he has done because he has wished or desired it. As a whole, mankind has considered desirable the transformation of energy from physical into mental. The basis of this desire is the greater mobility and versatility of mental over physical powers. Physical powers are exceedingly limited, limited in fact to the use of a comparatively few muscles, while mental powers are unlimited. It is as if a small amount of iron physical power could by the alchemy of education be transmuted into an enormous amount of golden mental power, and the feeling of superiority of the individual in whom this transmutation takes place is very gratifying to him, enabling him to overcome his fellows, and therein satisfying one of his fundamental cravings.

The craving to be active mentally is instinctive only in that sphere of thinking which is called undirected thinking or day-dreaming. That is a variety of mental activity which, however, is quite unconcerned with any positive effect upon external reality. A child or an adult will day-dream for hours, with no present and no future result, except that in a very small minority of cases an adult will dream constructively, will think out a plan of action or the plot of a story, and later the action will be carried out or the story will be written. Generally, however, day-dreaming is the only actual fulfilment of the unconscious wishes which are the really instinctive mental activity. Its essential characteristic is its practical futility, and the gradual change which it produces on the day-dreamer, making him less and less interested in real life and more and more centred upon himself, his mental eye being turned in towards his own thoughts and away from real things. An excessive introversion of this kind is seen in the form of insanity known as *dementia praecox.*

The motives for a change from the instinctive day-dreaming, which is natural, to what is apparently un-natural have to be kept clearly in view, or the whole educational procedure seems at once irrational. The main motive for the transfer from physical to mental activity, and from the undirected to a directed form of thinking, is really a better adjustment of the physical activity and not, as many have seemed to think, the reduction in amount or complete abolition of physical activity. We are primarily physical as well as mental, and the only real gain to civilization by means of mental improvement is an improvement of the physical condition.

The Physical Child

Now, the physical condition of the child is not a thing apart from his mental condition; it is not a separate thing which can be specially trained quite without regard to the mental state. If that were so, children could be put into mechanical exercisers, and their natural resistance would, in a reasonable time, produce a result of muscular physique which would delight the soul of the most materialistic trainer whose photographs of gnarly backs and lumpy arms one occasionally sees in shop windows and magazine advertisements. Extreme muscular strength is an attainable, but is not a desirable, aim. So a mild amount of mentality is injected into the physical training in the schools in the shape of games, dances, etc. And into the English study there is also injected a small amount of physical training in the shape of declamation and dramatics.

But this is practically all. Nor would it be possible to combine Latin and physical training or any other subject called cultural with physical training in the modes in which they appear in the school curriculum. The combination of physical and mental in the cultural subjects is there nevertheless, but in a much more subtle and elusive state; for the connection between the cultural subjects and the physical condition of the pupil is mediated solely by the unconscious, about which practically nothing is known by the average teacher.

It is quite common for the interest which is displayed by a child in a subject such as arithmetic to be the outward manifestation of a real though unconscious interest in the teacher. It would seem that this is not only possible but probable in all cases even where, as it is in some, the interest in the teacher is not consciously known. We do hear pupils say they like a study because they like the teacher of it. And we are all well acquainted with the pupils who cannot make head or tail out of a subject because the teacher is inferior. It would seem that a personally attractive teacher could arouse enthusiasm in a student for any subject whatever, whether or not the teacher knew anything about it at all.

The Unconscious Wish as a Tension

The aspect of the unconscious which influences the physical health of the pupil, as well as his mental health, is the unconscious wish. It has been shown by the newer psychology that the unconscious wish is a tension which is expressed only through the muscles, not only the larger and more familiar ones but also the very small ones of which we are never conscious. These small ones contract and expand with the result of enlarging and diminishing the calibre of the passages in the body through which go air, food, blood and various other fluids, and therefore govern the development of those parts of the physical organism which are supplied by the various chemical products of food, air and water.

These wishes or tensions or infinitesimal inceptive movements of the muscles are at once too small to enter our conscious life and yet so numerous and so powerful as to influence it greatly, though in ways that appear to be extremely indirect. They are, in their gross effects, distantly comparable with the rising or falling of the tide in a river which lifts a vessel alongside of a wharf, imperceptible to the eye while the eye has the patience to keep looking, and yet causing a change which is noticeable from time to time as one observes the height of the vessel against the wharf.

The wishes or tensions which exist unconsciously in the mind of every child when confronted with a school task of any nature whatsoever correspond, in this comparison, to the limitless force of the uplift of the water on the hull of the vessel, and the conscious attitude of the child corresponds to the physical effort which a boy or a girl might exert to oppose or assist in the upward movement of the boat on a rising tide. The effect on the boat is virtually nothing, while the effect on the boy or girl is directly in proportion to the effort put forth. Very wise are they if they cease exerting themselves as soon as they have stirred up a vigorous circulation.

And yet, some of the tasks assigned in school work are, if taken too seriously—that is, literally,—as hopeless as a single child's attempt to lift a thousand-ton vessel, or push it down into the water. The tasks, hopeless as they are, continue to be set, however, by teachers and devisers of curricula, and the inevitable result follows. Is anything except mental gymnastics accomplished, even though a full-rigged ship is put in the place of a dumb-bell? It is much as if one encouraged a pupil to make believe he was lifting the heavier weight, and gaining much glory from the fancied accomplishment, just because it is enormous. Of course, if they really could lift such a weight, they would be wonders. But we know they cannot, and they know they cannot, and so we practise them in the art of deceiving themselves and trying to deceive us.

It is not a mere matter of qualitative uncongeniality. The intellectual feats necessary to accomplish the mentally impossible they would gladly, many of them, perform, just as feats, to show power, but they soon realize the impossibility of doing them well, even when they pass examinations at 95% and 100%. What must be the real candid feeling of the graduate who has received above 90% on a paper in any subject? Not that the mark is a mark applicable to the subject, but that it is applicable to the person, who is, in truth, most inadequate to give a 90% account of the subject.

What, then, would be the result of giving to the pupils in secondary schools, or to the students in colleges, tasks that are commensurate with their comparatively slight abilities? The pride of the adults who are superintending the education of the adolescents would be severely hurt. To please our own fancy, to tickle our own imaginations, we pretend that the young people can handle Shakespeare, or Vergil, or chemistry or history or philosophy. And they, in their turn, are brought up to practise the same deception on *their* children when they come along and have to be educated.

Now, in all this hypocrisy the wishes for real accomplishment, the tensions or inceptive movements in the direction of attaining ends really and not imaginatively attainable, are bound to be frustrated. The young would really like to do what they can to help along civilization and well-being of every kind. For the unconscious wish is always a wish for power and for life. And when the conscious mind of the person being educated in schools is faced with a task which, if taken literally, is impossible, only the child-power of the *conscious* life is really enlisted, and not the race-power of the *unconscious*. In all this fruitless struggle, the unconscious, which is comparable to a different personality residing in the same body as the conscious personality, is perfectly aware of the futility of the efforts which are being put forth by the consciousness, and does not share in them, for it must by nature strive for *results* which are the resolutions of the tensions making up its essence.

The unconscious is one continued wish or tension or bundle of tensions. These tensions are relaxed or resolved naturally from time to time in the act of creating or the act of eating. I use the word creating instead of reproduction, for the reason that the two main forms of the desire perpetuation are the perpetuation of self, and, as a variety of self-perpetuation, that of the race. Now, the race-perpetuating instinct, like all instincts springing from it, is transmutable. It may be transmuted from one kind of creation to another. This transformation of the creative instinct from physical reproduction of species to production or creation of other things, which has always been spoken of as higher, is called by the aspiring name of sublimation. And it is really higher from the point of view of personal power and accomplishment. For the difficulties overcome in accomplishing it, which measure the value of it as a conscious production, are much greater than in the reproduction of kind, in which one acts spontaneously, without resistance and without sense of personal achievement or with only an illusory one. What nature causes and completes is so separate from the Ego, that opposes and overcomes that nature in us, that our overcoming it seems much more our own doing than anything in which nature wholly concurs. Thus it is evident that the accomplishment most gratifying to the individual consciousness is that which most overcomes, masters or controls the instinctive and unconscious tendencies. In yielding to and falling in with the instincts, which are absolutely common and universal, we are not developing that power which most typifies our existence as individuals. In doing the most common things we are surrendering our separateness as individuals and sinking ourselves into a larger organism—the race.

Reproductive vs. Productive Creation

The primal urge or generic expression of vitality which keeps alive the living things on earth shows itself in mankind as the driving force which prolongs the individual life and propagates the species. This purely propagative desire I will call desire for *reproductive* creation, and distinguish it from its more refined form which might be called *productive* creation. Whenever the craving to create, which is the fundamental one in all humanity, is raised by any circumstances whatever into an urge to create not the reduplication of the self in other individuals, offspring (which I call reproductive creation because it merely repeats units like those which already exist), but to create something new in the world by the manipulation of real things already existent into a new production which never existed before, such as a house or a book or a picture, I would call this latter kind of creation productive. Education is aimed solely at productive creation, though it is unfortunately true that instinct alone is not enough properly to direct the other kind. Left undirected, reproductive creation is, in the majority of cases, the cause of much misery which education in the distant future will, I am sure, contribute much to remove from the world.

Every idea which occurs to us is a manifestation of the unconscious wish for creation, whether it be that continued creation of self which is otherwise called self-preservation, or that intermittent creation of other personalities called reproduction. There is no idea that is not originally caused to come into consciousness by that primal urge. This seems a very extraordinary statement when we apply it to the idle fancies or chance associations which occasionally come into our heads. Why, when I am writing these words, does a picture suddenly flash before my mental eye, a picture of a piece of road in Vermont over which I drove two summers ago? I do not know positively, and could not be sure unless I spent a great deal of time studying other idle and apparently chance and trivial associations which might occur to me during the three or four hours which I might devote to the investigation this evening. Why, when I am reading Sully's " Pessimism," do I get another mental picture, extremely vivid, of a convivial scene under the trees, with tables and a luncheon served on them and a group of people having a jolly time? I surmise in this case that the tenor of the pessimism book evoked in me an opposing wish to be optimistic, and that this wish took the form of a banquet in an orchard, a bright visualization, which was the only medium then available for the unconscious to express a wish which might be put in the words: " I wish I were feasting on real food instead of purely mental pabulum, on delicious viands instead of on dry philosophic bones, and with a company of jolly people instead of alone, in the open air at noon instead of in a stuffy room at midnight."

Occurrence of Thoughts or Actions

An exceedingly important fact to realize is that every slightest thought coming into anyone's head is, so to speak, the visible form of the primal urge which has caused him to be here and alive today and has caused the existence of every living thing that has ever come into being. It seems to be exceedingly important both for his present and his future and important in its bearing upon education.

In the first place its enormous importance in education lies in the fact that it clears up a great many doubtful points as to the applicability of different types of education, technical, cultural, etc., as to the actual methods of presentation to the pupil and as to the relation existing between pupil and teacher. It explains much more clearly the necessity for the teacher and the teacher's work, and accounts for much of the strained relation which exists between teacher and student. Not only every slightest and most trivial idea which occurs either to student or teacher, but every littlest act of either of them, is causally connected with their own unconscious wishes for creativeness. The string of intermediate causes between a disorderly pupil's unconscious desire to accomplish, in the world, work of a concrete effectualness and his disorderly conduct in breaking a piece of furniture, losing or destroying a book, or diverting the attention of the entire classroom to himself by means of some exhibitionistic act—the string of intermediate causes between the individual pupil's disorder and the cosmic order which actuates his unconscious desires, is sometimes very long and complicated. It is in every strand's length connected by his reasoning faculty with his relations to fellow-student and teacher—a causal connection which has never, I believe, been taken into consideration in planning any educational work, for the reason that never until the present time has it been recognized.

Up to the present time the association of ideas has been

regarded as a chance affair, a purely accidental matter, for which no laws could be discovered. Similarly the restless actions, apparently aimless, the multitudinous blunders, omissions and mistakes committed in school or college work have up to date been regarded as accidents. But just as the word "accident" (coming from two Latin words meaning "a falling toward," of one body in the direction of another) from a modern scientific viewpoint implies an attraction exerted by the one body upon the other, so in modern psychology we must suppose the existence of a force determining the occurrence of an idea, of an idea to do a thing and just as much the existence of a force causing an action which is not accompanied by an idea (a so-called automatic action) as so many actions are, both of adults and children.

I say an action not accompanied by an idea. Of course I mean an action not accompanied by an idea of which we are conscious. The idea may nevertheless be in the unconscious, a notion which is the newer psychology's contribution to the theory of education. And just as I have occasion to say elsewhere that every emotion is connected with an idea, so here I say that every act is connected with a thought, although that thought may or may not be in consciousness at the time. We rightly speak of thoughtless acts, if we mean that such acts are not, at manifestation, accompanied by the appropriate conscious thoughts. But on careful consideration it is quite evident that an action is but the outward manifestation of a thought, sometimes a thought which has crossed the threshold from the unconscious into consciousness, but often a thought which remains in the unconscious. The expression "thoughtless acts," then, fitly represents this condition, which is a very striking one, and seems at first sight very extraordinary if not impossible. But what is a thoughtless act if not an act which has been caused by a thought that does not exist in consciousness, to be sure, but does exist in the unconscious part of the personality of the thoughtless actor?

Thoughtless Acts

So we should be very careful to keep clear the true implication of the thoughtless acts of children or adults. Very frequently both act thoughtlessly, but the thoughtlessness is only in the comparatively narrow sphere of consciousness. The thought itself which gave form to the act yet lives, but it lives and moves and has its being in that illimitable world of the unconscious; the thought causing your thoughtless act lives in your unconscious, and the thought causing my thoughtless act lives in my unconscious, and so on for every person in the world.

As soon as we have clearly seen this very definite fact of the rigid natural causation between thought and act, between conscious thought and conscious act, between conscious act and conscious thought, relations which have always been recognized, and between conscious act and unconscious thought, between unconscious act and unconscious thought and between unconscious thought and unconscious act, relations which are only now beginning to be recognized, we shall see also the connection between unconscious thought and those varieties of act which are partly conscious and partly unconscious. By this I mean errors, blunders, mistakes of all kinds, slips of the pen, tongue, hand, foot, etc., none of which has hitherto had any *significance* for teacher or pupil, but which now are seen to have a very deep one. For it is a fact amply demonstrated that every error is the partly unconscious gratification of an unconscious wish, and as all unconscious wishes are wishes for one or the other kind of creativeness, it turns out paradoxically enough that the so-called accidental breaking of an object or the tearing of a page or the spoiling of a written exercise is the conscious manifestation of an unconscious wish to create and not to destroy. This fact puts a different aspect upon all the misdeameanours of children and makes understandable in a way never before appreciated the words: Forgive them, for they know not what they do.

Organ Inferiority Naturally Compensated

A defence of the present system of education is that it gives a well-rounded development, that the subjects which the student finds disagreeable or difficult are the very ones he most needs, inasmuch as his disinclination to follow them up is an indication that they are his weak points, and that if he should be allowed to neglect them he would be like a person refusing to exercise his weak arms and preferring to develop further his comparatively strong legs. It is also a fact, on the other hand, that an innate constitutional weakness in any part of the organism tends to be compensated for, not merely by a greater strengthening of some other part, as when a blind man develops keener sense of touch than one who sees normally, but in many cases the constitutional weakness or inferiority of an organ, such as an eye, results in a more efficient use and greater development of the same organ, as when a person with low sensitivity to colour or form becomes, by this compensating mechanism, an artist, or one with a constitutional defect of hearing becomes a musician. That is to say, the unconscious, perceiving the defect of the organ in question, devotes a greater part of its power to the perfection of the functioning of the inferior organ than the unconscious of a person in whom no such defect exists, and in whom of course that organ will remain forever unnoticed. Thus the classical illustration of the difficulty of this nature triumphantly overcome is that of Demosthenes, who conquered an impediment in his speech with so great an impetus that he became an orator. And in our own day there are numberless illustrations of the same, of which I might mention the case of Annette Kellerman, the great swimmer, who is said to have been, as a child, delicate and unusually afraid of the water.*

So that the argument that the natural bent of a person is not the thing to be developed because it is his strong point, and the so-called faculties he shows no interest in developing are his weak points, is really based on a misinterpretation of the facts. One is most sensitive about his weak points and essentially what one takes the most interest in is the element in his mental or physical make-up which is the tenderest and most sensitive, so that one's natural bent is towards one's inferior faculty; and if education is to do the best for the individual, it should help him develop his weak point, feeling assured that what he takes least interest in he has least to fear from.

---

* If a rubber automobile tire tube is inflated, the thinner spots expand the most, the weaker parts are the ones to swell up to the greater size from the pressure of the air within.

It is evident that a perfectly functioning part attracts no attention. We never know we have a stomach until we have indigestion. We never know where our *appendix vermiformis* is (or was) until disorders in certain locations call our conscious attention thither, and, in some cases, make the defects our strongest points. Similarly we, as a race, must have thought or felt that our mentality was our weak point judging from the hysterical efforts we have made to fortify that position by academic education.

There is another consideration which comes in here. If Gerald or Gladys has a perfectly good mathematical head and can do twice as much as Betty or Bobby, they of course to a certain extent enjoy the prestige which this superiority gives them and will more or less take advantage of the opportunity for exhibitionism of a mild type which they have, but the prominence thus gained is made uncomfortable for them frequently by the remarks only quasi-admiring which their companions and relatives make about them at school and at home. In short, there is in every domestic and scholastic environment a mild tendency to look upon mathematical excellence, at least, as a sort of freakishness. The boy or girl who can work without effort the most exacting algebraic problems arouses in other pupils and even to a certain extent in the adults of the environment a certain degree of envy which is expressed in one of two ways, commonly. It is expressed as extravagant compliment, the insincerity of which is quite apparent to the victim of it, or it comes out as a statement that those who excel in mathematics generally do not excel in anything else. This, if repeated often enough to constitute a family tradition, has a very suggestive effect upon the child who suffers from such remarks.

Then there is in a great many people, young and old, an unfortunate tendency to belittle the accomplishments in which they themselves excel and to overvalue the accomplishments of others. This has both a subjective and an objective cause. The objective cause is the very fact that misery loves company and that those who are inexpert in anything have many sympathizers. They have lots of good company. The subjective cause is found in the fact that a very great many young people have numerous good but unconscious reasons for not wishing to excel in anything. Excellence brings responsibilities, as riches provoke appeals. One who can do anything superlatively well has many requests to perform, both for the profitless exhibition of his prowess and, as numberless people in all walks of life will testify, for the actual doing of favours from which the recipient is the only person to benefit. It is only recently that the doctrine of selling oneself to all people in a certain sense is being advocated as the best means of getting on. It is quite evident on careful consideration that this preparing of oneself to serve others and in so doing correctly evaluating one's own powers has no small part to play in the unconscious life, if it has not in the conscious life of even the very young school child.

What are, then, the activities, mental and physical, which will enlist the unconscious wishes as well as the conscious ones, and enable the incipient motions to be carried out to an end which shall be the appropriate relaxation of the tension? For every tension aims only at relaxation or resolution and every state of relaxation must, for life to continue, be followed by a tension. So a rhythm is set up which is the rhythm of life. A mass of protoplasm absolutely relaxed would be a spineless, nerveless and therefore motionless body which would never subsequently move of itself. So that in the relaxed tissues, mental and physical, after the discharge of the activity, there must be a nucleus of a new tension, an embryonic wish which is to be the father of the new tension; or else a part of the old wish must be left as the beginning of the new one, in which case the discharge of energy producing the relaxation would not be complete each time. Possibly an absolutely complete discharge would be synonymous with death.

We have seen that if the activities proposed for the child do not enlist the coöperation of the unconscious wish, there is never a real accomplishment, but only a pretended one, and if it is not thought that the pretended accomplishments are not as good as the real ones, it will seem necessary to chose the *real* accomplishments for the young and set them the task of achieving the real things of life. Now, what are the tasks that can be set for children to accomplish as something really valuable to society?

The only thing accomplished by the effort to lift a ship was the heating of the individual's body who tried. The only effect of the effort to master the meaning of Shakespeare or Vergil or Napier or Lavoisier is the wearing of grooves in the brain of the child. On the other hand, the only result worth attaining by mortals is a result effected upon the external world. This is true both because of the effect on the world and the effect on the individual. They are both different. The only result attained by a great many people is a resulting change in themselves by virtue of which they react to the world in a manner different from the way they did. This is the only result gained by the present system of education from the kindergarten to the doctorate. It may be said that the full course of twenty years of education *may* be *preparing* the young person to follow some calling when it calls, though there is a great of diversity of opinion about this point. We never shall be able to tell whether it does or not, because we never shall know how the boy who has gone through college would have done if he had not gone, and our own testimony about ourselves is worthless.

Turning the Child from Reality

Is the change to which we subject the children for twenty years in schools and colleges a real change and a desirable change? I believe that up to the present time the only essential change has been an undesirable one. What we have really accomplished in the youth of our country is a turning them away from reality.

There have been many motives for turning children away from reality, the same motives we have ourselves for turning away from reality, motives which may be grouped under the one rubric—undesirability. To consciousness of a certain type and at a certain stage of development reality is undesirable because it is bad or unpleasant. It is hard, it is unsympathetic, hostile, it is ugly, and fatiguing, and it smells bad. In contrast to this ideality is everything that reality is not. Heaven is the mental projection of everything that is idealized, the product of a phantasy compensating for the sense of inferiority, of lack of mastery, of misery in general, which a certain type of humanity experiences in its contact with the world.

Just as the infant annihilates an uncomfortable sensation with a wriggle or represses the pangs of hunger by the ecstatic sucking on its thumb, so do adults annihilate the adversities of an objective world by a mental wriggle, and repress the pangs of unsatisfied desire of all kinds by ecstatic absorption in an ideal vision or phantasy. If we have not what we think we want, we can get it ideally by vivid imagination. In *A Kiss for Cinderella,* little " Miss Thing " wishes so hard, in order to balance her unhappy lot, that she succeeds in a dream in imagining a ball exactly as she would desire it.

This turning away from reality is inevitable when the mental content of the person is words rather than ideas or things. The use of money as a medium of exchange of goods is analogous to the use of words as a means of exchange of ideas (=things=goods). The special attention to money as such makes the numismatist or the bank teller or the miser. The special attention to words as such makes the philologist or the lexicographer or the lunatic.

We cannot give our boys and girls practical experience in geography by sending them from one country to another. Some of them take it themselves by running away, and of these many make very fine men. Those not so fine are not less fine solely on account of their travels and experience of the world, but for other reasons.

We cannot give our boys and girls practical experience in the household arts. Only a few get it, and the number is diminishing yearly. An attempt to make up for it is being made by the schools with courses in sewing and domestic science. But the actual time that is devoted to this activity is so short and the results are so meagre that they can be ignored.

We cannot as a *part* of a school course adequately train young people to be stenographers and typewriters. We cannot, in short, make of them valuable operatives or workers of any kind while they are in school or college. If they turn out to be good workers, it is in spite of their school tasks, and not because of them. What, then, do we do with them in our educational institutions? We do two things to their unconscious wishes. We repress their unconscious wishes to do *real* things in the world, for there is no real thing done in school. I have been many times mildly disgusted with the universal attitude of boys and girls toward the visible result of their school work, results visible in the shape of exercises in algebra, English, French, Latin. Naturally, of course, they throw them away, as soon as they think the teacher's eye is finally removed from them. And I myself in earnest zeal collected notes in college, thinking I might use them some time, but I have never once had occasion to refer to them. The student knows that every word he writes, every sum he does, every exercise he finishes has been done and repeatedly done by millions of other children. Every fact imparted to him in biology, for instance, is better expressed and more beautifully illustrated in numberless inexpensive manuals, any one of which could be gotten on almost an hour's notice, if he had

any use for it.   There is in this kind of prescribed work
a sort of double uselessness for the student.   If he did
it as well as a school child or a college man could possibly do it, there is a multitude of other forms in which
the same work has been done and all of them as good or
better.

I emphasize this point in order to bring out the fact
that one of the main unconscious wishes is here in every
child frustrated, namely the wish for superiority, and I
am sure that the wish for superiority, for mastery, for
victory, is a wish for a real mastery over the external
world and not a mastery of self.   And this victory over
the external world is rendered impossible by waging the
battle in a place immured from the world, in the school
(=schola=leisure=absence of real work), and the high-
school pupils take for their graduating motto *Ex scholae
vita in scholam vitae,** which fitly symbolizes the segregation.   Thus are the main unconscious wishes inevitably
frustrated.   It is agreed, by common consent of all
parties, of pupils, teachers and parents, that the work
of the schools and colleges *cannot* of itself be really
productive.

But I do not believe that the most educative activity,
that which draws out of a man or woman the best that
is in him or her, can possibly be an activity which represses the unconscious desire to do real things, acomplish
real results, create real new entities, which in the real
world every real worker is doing from the labourer to
the banker, from the switchman to the railroad pres-
ident(?).

If we should say to a child, "You've *got* to play till

* Out from the life of school into the school of life.

you're twenty-five; you've *got* to make believe till you're a full-grown man," he would revolt at the thought, for even the play of the most real children is an imitation of the real activities they see about them. They want to be policemen, firemen, engineers, storekeepers, they consciously desire to do the very things they see adults do, and the system of education handed down from antiquity represses their conscious desires for concrete reality into their unconscious, it continues this repression for twenty years in some cases, requiring them to accept words in place of things, symbols in lieu of the realities academically symbolized.

Possible Reality in Child's Life

And what are the real things which, in spite of the academic barriers designed apparently to keep real things out,—what are the real things which the boy or girl gets in the artificial life of school or college? For they do, in spite of their immurement, get *some* reality. A common distinction is made between lessons, lectures, tasks, exercise, etc., and the school or college " activities " which we all know are quite the opposite in character, but are academicized in order to fit into the system. They get football and basket-ball and societies and dances, and the boys and girls get each other, which is no doubt very good for them. They get to know each other better, but for this they have not to thank the teachers or superintendents or the system in general. They are face to face with reality in the shape of each other, but a reality toned down and made constrained and artificial by the aggressive presence of teachers and equipment.

I said that the unconscious wishes of the student are repressed in two ways, by the suppression of the wish for superiority, which can be satisfied only on concrete reality, and there is another which I have not mentioned. It is the substitution for it of a highly artificial system of unrealities, the net result of which on the student is an unconscious or partly conscious impression of hypocrisy, deception and insincerity. Even in the ancient Roman times whence all this pedagoguery originated, Juvenal satirized the senselessness of the school children arguing about supposititious problems.

I am aware that I seem to verge toward realism and away from idealism (the ideal being the consequently superior), and invite the uncomplimentary comments of all who deem themselves idealistic and aspiring to higher ideals, the life of reason as opposed to the life of passion, the intellectual as opposed to the material, and I shall by thoughtless ones be branded as a crass materialist. But I feel that the concept of the development of the mind-body combination which I shall propose is as truly idealistic as possibly could be, and at the same time remain practical.

For I think the time will some day come when children will be taught to do what they can constructively and creatively accomplish. We proceed today upon the principle that an individual cannot actually produce any valuable work until he is about twenty-five years old, whereas we know that physical puberty comes to men as early as fourteen and women as early as twelve. We thus keep from productive work some women until ten or twelve years after they are physically capable of maternity, and some men for almost as many years are kept from creative work. In other words, dominated by the analogy between the comparatively greater length of the period of infancy in humans than in other animals, we consciously and purposely attempt to lengthen the period of adolescence, thinking thereby to make an added improvement. We have thought to improve the adulthood by keeping the young people adolescent as long as possible, because kittens and chickens who can forage for themselves after a very brief period of maternal care are not highly spiritual beings. We have gone on the principle that, in order to fit the individual best to fight the battle of real life, we should keep him from battle as long as possible, as if the best preparation for any activity was assiduously *not* doing that very thing, as if the deepest knowledge of any object were gained by carefully keeping the individual isolated from that object, so that he could not hear, see, touch or exercise any of his senses upon it.

Early Acquaintance with Reality

I am convinced that the best preparation for the world reality that can be given for the child from the earliest moment when it can dispense with personal maternal care, is actual concrete acquaintance with the realities of the world, and furthermore that every generation of humans has been prepared for its later experiences of life solely by means of the earlier experiences of the same life, and that, too, in spite of any organized attempt to imprison him in schools.

Is it impossible that children should be unable to do *any* productive work as soon as they can handle simple tools? I believe that the training which the child can get in natural surroundings in a rural district in touch with the animal and vegetable world is the training which best fits him to cope later with the various emergencies of human existence. That this is not the uniform result in the case of country-bred youth I admit, but I think it is the fault of the human element in the country and not the nature element.

As the tendency is for children born and bred in the country to go to the city, so there should be a reciprocal tendency of city-born children to go to the country. If it is reasonable for a human to desire every kind of experience, those in the city and in the country should change places. In the country a child can be productive at a very early age in doing things for which only vision and locomotion are necessary, such as herding various animals and later in caring for them when the children become strong enough. In the city too there is plenty of real work that children could do, if it were only permitted. I am not arguing for child-labour, which means excessive toil such as tending for wearisome hours the cotton machines in the South, but for a moderate amount of child activity which may be encouragingly productive for the child. In the country the work done by the child has the courage taken out of it through being unrewarded by selfish parents, whence comes the spiritual impossibility of it.

Some parents will say, "Let the children help their parents." In the country boys can and do help their fathers, and to a limited extent in the city. And both boys and girls can help around the house. But it is notorious how much they prefer to help in other people's houses rather than helping their own families. In the first place they are, in helping other people than their own families, doing something of their own accord, and in the second they are much more generously rewarded in praise and other more material ways than at home, where their services are taken as a matter of course and as something due. Then there is the variety, which has a great appeal for everyone, not only children. I remember as a boy leaving my own small garden uncared for, which my mother declared she could not understand, and going to work for the farmers in the neighbourhood.

Is a young person's recreation a bit less wholesome, if it comes after a brief period of actual creation of value? Because all work and no play makes Jack dull, are we to deprive him of all work? Work and play, child and man, city and country, travel and home should all be mingled in about equal proportions, so that everyone could have some of everything.

True Democracy in Education

This will in some distantly future day work out in somewhat the following manner, when there is true democracy and political and every other kind of equality. Children will be taken over from the parents to the state between the ages of five and ten years. If city born they will be transferred to the country, and vice versa, at a later date. They will be sent to different parts of the country, too, and engage in different occupations in all of which they will take huge delight. They will share in all the occupations of adults, and will keep moving in circuits from place to place, returning occasionally to their own parents, but in the meantime living with other children's parents in other homes. The children in each house will change periodically, thus giving the adults a new experience, as well as themselves. Each child will be required to keep a diary, which he or she will read to each new household, as they progress through the land, and thus the necessary practice in verbal training will be given. The homes thus exchanged will be kept up to a standard of efficiency and morale by government inspectors, and the hours of work, recreation and study will be regulated according to the best interests of the world-nation for the production of the most useful citizens.

There will be no hermits. Every social duty which should be performed by everyone will be performed by everyone. Everyone will have the widest possible variety of experience, including work, recreation and solitude, noise, music and silence, action and inaction in properly distributed proportions. There will not only be no actual ostensible hermits but there will be no spiritual hermits of the repressed variety. Everybody's mind will be open to everybody else's inspection, just as now everybody's face in Caucasian countries is open, and not veiled up to the eyes. Only when we shall finally be able to look the whole world in the face, not alone because we owe not any man but because or in spite of the fact that we do owe or have been guilty, or have failed, shall we be able to live in a really social atmosphere, and develop all the relations which alone evoke the fullest growth in ourselves. In this more conscious illumined time to which I am now looking forward, when people shall have crawled forth from the egotistical prison cells in which they are now benighted—" Confined and pestered in this pinfold here "—true superiority will be recognized and repression of the kind which drives unpleasant or painful ideas back into the unconscious will not exist. Anybody may say or attempt to do anything to anybody, and no offence can be taken, because an insult, for instance, will be unable to act as a complex-indicator in the person insulted, but only in the insulting person, provided that so much unwholesomeness remains as to render such waste of time possible. A person who insults another because he himself has done a wrong will be illuminated sufficiently to see that it is his own maladjustment which he is verbally expressing, and not the action of the insulted person.

A Recitation Experiment

At the present time, and with educational facilities limited as they are, it is of course impracticable to attempt any of the innovations suggested above for the purpose of making the child's life more real. But the teacher in the school of the present day can reproduce to some extent the mental attitudes of adults in the world without the school. Even in such a subject so far removed from the present day as an ancient language, the method of handling the required work can be approximated to the spiritual environment which the child will find outside of the school. It may be said that the teacher is in complete control of the situation in the classroom in his ability to reproduce through his actions the atmosphere which the child will meet in the world or to create a cloister-like atmosphere which will make the child's entrance into the world an entrance into an entirely strange place in which he will not know how to act.

With a view to reproducing in his classroom some of the elements of the real extra-academic conditions a teacher of Latin in one of the high schools of a large city instituted a scheme which he found to work very well. Its essential feature was the instant recognition of and immediate recompense for the mental activity of the pupil. It was to a certain degree modelled upon the old-fashioned spelling bee. Seating the members of the class at the beginning of the term in a chance order (alphabetical), he allowed the first pupil in the class, as thus arranged, to recite first. If his recitation was defective in the slightest degree, the next pupil was given the chance to do the same thing. If he did it perfectly, he changed places with the first pupil. The actual shifting about was found to be an immense relief to the pupils, and legitimately released a great deal of physical energy which is superfluous at that age. The chance to " recite " passed down the whole class, giving an equal opportunity to each pupil to express himself in his best manner, which he con-stantly studied by comparison with the mistakes of others. When a pupil at the head of the class made a perfect recitation he went to the foot of the class and had the opportunity to make his way again to the head. Each complete progress through the class was recorded by the teacher, and the relative accomplishments of all the pupils were on record, and available for report at any time according to their positions in the class and the number of times they had gone from the foot to the head. The similarity of the situation to extra-mural reality is twofold, for the child can by this means get an immediate reward for his attention and his effort and he can plan by preparation for more distant ends and aims. At the end of one day's recitation each pupil's position in the class is registered by the fact that he is represented by a card, and the cards can either be collected or handed in by the pupils in the exact position in which they were at the end of the period. At the beginning of the next day's recitation the cards are laid on the desks in the order in which they were taken up and the game goes on at exactly the point where it was interrupted. There is thus a continuity which is preserved for a whole term.

A word should be said as to just what is meant by a " recitation." It can mean any unit of expression, great or small, which the teacher finds it best to use. For instance, in beginners' Latin classes a " recitation " means the inflection of the singular of a noun, or the reading and translation of a short sentence of Latin. In third-year Latin it may mean the translation of a paragraph of Cicero, or a sentence or a clause, according to the exigencies of the case. It may mean the translation of a sentence from English into Latin, or the statement concerning the syntax of a noun or a verb.

In order to correlate the attention of all the pupils, the teacher invites the criticism of each and every one. Anyone having a criticism to make raises his hand, and at the proper time is recognized by the teacher, exactly as a member of a deliberative assembly is recognized by the chair. If the criticism is just, the pupil making it is allowed to go ahead of the one sitting ahead of him, who

takes the inferior place. Any suggestion on the part of
the pupils about any point connected with the work is
accepted by the " chair," but if it is ruled out as being
a bad one, in any way unsocial, as obstructing the work
in hand rather than furthering it, the maker of the suggestion is fined by being required to go back one place.
Thus is secured a high degree of flexibility, a true democracy, and a focussing of attention on the work to be done.
The conduct of the recitation is in the hands of the
pupils themselves, and it is sometimes inspiring to see
the intensity of interest that is manifested, each pupil
trying his best to improve his position in the class by
studying the performances of the others. So tense was
the atmosphere on one occasion, so breathlessly did the
class as a whole watch the performance of a particularly
good student that the ticking of a small clock in a closet
in the classroom was quite audible. The details of this
scheme are so interesting, so close to the unconscious
wish for superiority does it bring even the work connected with a dead language, that the pupils have themselves made many suggestions which have been adopted,
materially changing certain features of it, and, I am
told, it is in a continual process of evolution.

The " work " of the teacher, as regards details which
are purely academic and non-social, is reduced to a minimum. On the principle that the pupils are the ones who
should develop themselves, and that the teacher should
not be the only one whose mind is to be improved, the
expressions of personality are almost entirely on the part
of the pupils. The teacher could leave the class and the
work go on in his absence, almost as well, after the class
as a whole has grasped the main idea of it. In this sense

it is highly democratic, social and progressive. There is no theme which may not come up in connection with the work and be treated with the utmost ability of any of the members of the class. The lecturing tendency of the teacher is properly reduced, and the points are brought out by the individual activities of the pupils. It has been a continual surprise and delight on the part of the teacher to see how many new points of view the pupils, in this scheme, have the confidence to bring out, and this teacher believes that the dead language Latin, handled in this way, is much more alive than some of the biology which is taught in the ordinary method.

While the strictly administrative work of the teacher is reduced to a minimum by this developing method of conducting a recitation, his duties of guide and adviser are much increased because he has to meet new situations continually. The relations of the topics connected with the life of today are real and not artificial. Not only in the Cicero classes is the parallel between present conditions and those at Rome in the days of the conspiracy brought out by the pupils themselves, according to their observation of the life of today as they get it out of school, but in the lower classes there is a special means of making the schoolroom environment much more like that of the world which the pupil will later enter. The teacher in short reacts to the expressions of the pupils in exactly the same way, wherever possible, in which the people whom the pupils would meet with the greatest advantage to themselves would act toward them.

A great resistance is manifested to the conditions of this scheme by the pupils who are unable to face the

adversities of the world. It is very much like a defeat
and in some children least able to cope with the world
arouses a deep resentment at first to be required to go
back and physically and literally give way before a superior. His inferiority is " rubbed in " in a very unpleasant
manner—at first, until he finds that he can by his own
efforts recover the position he has lost. But once having
found out how quick are the rewards for his sincere efforts, how instantly he can produce an effect with them, he
realizes that he has it in his power to place himself as high
in the class as he wishes.

The experience of this teacher with this scheme of
eliciting the expressions of the individuality of the pupil
has shown him that the unit of expression is very small
at first and that it gradually increases in scope. For instance, in the teaching of Latin prose he has found that
a preparation was necessary in the minds of most pupils
for translating the English into Latin which they would
not themselves make unless they were put through it in a
regular manner—namely, the arrangement of the order
of the Latin words. The scheme of securing this developed into the following. The pupil first reciting a
sentence was required to rephrase the English in such a
way as to give the English words in the Latin order,
after which the next person gave a part or the whole of
the Latin translation. Thus " Caesar led his army out
of camp and drew it up " would have to be " meta-
phrased " as: " Caesar army from-camp having-been-
led-out drew-up." It turned out that the process was very
difficult at first but became quite easy later, and produced
in the pupil a much greater power of handling the Latin.
Then it developed that a very valuable result was secured

by giving the sentence to a number of pupils equal to the number of the Latin words in it, and getting each one to contribute one word, repeating what had been given before him. This produced a very keen attention on the part of the pupil, who realized that he had not only to remember what his predecessors had said, and attend to their pronunciation very carefully but that he had to be absolutely sure of what he was going to say, because on that sentence he would probably get only one chance. Furthermore, he never knew when he would be called on to recite, because he never could tell how many pupils ahead of him would fall down on some detail in the pronunciation or other feature of the performance.

Slowly and by a natural evolution this very simple scheme worked out into a great many complicated details, each pupil taking an interest in contributing some recommendation to help the scheme along as a social proceeding, although the words social or democratic were never used in the room. The scheme worked itself, became a living thing, because it appealed to a fundamental instinct of human nature, the same instinct which is the basis of all democratic government. It had the further result of giving to the pupils a feeling of control, which obviated the necessity of the teacher's asserting verbally his authority. In fact, it removed from the room the feeling which is unconsciously present in the mind of every pupil in the ordinary schoolroom, a feeling that he was acting under authority. It was gratifying to see how the infringements of the principle that all activity had to be helpful were not only paid for by the pupils' suggesting penalties for each other, but how frequently when a pupil had even unwittingly or forgetfully done anything

obstructive, he would go back one place, thus imposing
a fine upon himself for doing something which it is possible that no one but himself saw.

A democratic form of schoolroom management has
been introduced into some schools and labelled the
" school city." In each classroom a mayor is elected, a
police department, etc., with the court and trials and
other legal machinery, but it seems that this teacher's
scheme was far simpler and came much nearer to getting
at the real unconscious motives of the pupils.

Exceptionless Perfection of Nature

One is impressed with the tremendous unity of nature,
everything except man apparently completely fulfilling
its appointed function all the time without interruption.
Man alone seems to be interrupted, his development arrested, his perfection prevented. But we do see imperfect
things in nature, dwarfed, blasted trees and other apparent miscarryings. Yet they are as perfect as their
environment allows them to be. Are all humans as perfect as their surroundings permit? They must be. Are
there no perverse humans? Is there no wilful wrong?
There can be none, for why should we believe that natural laws work less perfectly in human than in plant or
animal life? Is not the most bestial human the best
product that his circumstances could make of him? Why
do we blame him for his inhuman condition? Is he not
taking, just as we take, the only steps possible to express
his power, to get his feeling of superiority, his control
over his environment?

Why Educate at All?

What, then, do we try to do in education? Improve on nature, whose laws are inexorable and perfect? Or is there some training which is superlatively human, which the uneducated lack and the academically educated receive? What the human gets by being trained in the specifically human traits is a development of his consciousness and one of the main objects of education is to bring into consciousness as many thoughts as possible in such a way as to give him a greater power over his surroundings. And this amplifying of the conscious life is not an increase of scope of consciousness at any given moment, but is, on the contrary, the individual's ability to bring into consciousness more of past experiences than he would naturally do if left to himself. For the natural man, without education, is limited in his scope of consciousness by the repressions which the fortuity of his environment imposes upon him. The uneducated man is a perfect and flawless effect of all the causes which determine him body and soul, but the educated man is the only one who has the power, however seldom he uses it, of altering his *psychical* environment.

Physical vs. *Psychical Environment*

Perhaps I will have to define what I mean by a psychical environment and differentiate it from a physical one. Any man can change his physical environment by, for instance, setting his house on fire, or by raising a field of potatoes, but in so doing he does not change his psychical environment, which is the way he mentally reacts to the physical ones, but by conscious effort along directed lines he can change his mode of psychical reaction to physical surroundings. He can change it from a passive, receptive one in which he follows the inexorable laws of nature in the same way that animals do, or he can acquire through directed thinking the only characteristic in which he can differ from the animals. His inherent difference from the lower orders consists in his *ability to acquire the greater amplitude of consciousness* referred to above. There is no doubt that the savage is little above the animal in this respect, and that the thoughts of the seer are as far removed as possible from the dim consciousness of the uncivilized, and that the general consensus of all men is that the seer's thoughts are more productive and have a wider influence than the savage's. Therefore society has created the seer and held him up as a goal toward which all men should aspire to attain and travel as far on the road thither as is possible. In creating this standard society has placed a greater value on conscious thoughts, so expressed that they can be reproduced in the minds of many people, than it has placed on any other human creation.

Amplifying the Consciousness

From this the consciousness-increasing aim of conscious education emerges clearly into view—to bring more things (or thoughts) into consciousness, but they must be thoughts of a certain kind, thoughts having in them enough of a quality common to all mankind to be accepted by all, and a further quality such that they inspire to action, also of a certain kind. The kind of action required is that which is for the common good, or for the attainment of social aims.

One of the advantages gained by the control over the mental reactions to physical environment is that a person having such control over himself is not harmed in the same way by the so-called adversities coming to him from the external world, and is not afraid to exert himself upon it. Much accomplishment that would be put through by people is prevented by their fear, either of their own inability to accomplish or of the harmful results which might come to them from pushing their efforts to the utmost.

Academic Education to Remove Unconscious Fear

The best academic education partially removes this fear, which is largely to blame for the failures of the youths and maidens who are being academically educated to accomplish the work laid out for them. But when we remember that all fear is unconsciously determined, we see that the person who because of fear does ill at school or college is the very one who will most be helped by acquiring this new knowledge. He is also the one who is dominated by fear outside of school.

When I say that all fear is unconsciously determined I mean that fear is really at bottom unconscious desire. A conscious fear of being unable to do a given lesson is really an unconscious desire to do it, and a state of mind in which fear is specially predominant, such as a phobia, is one where there is a strong desire (in the phobia fundamentally sexual) which is being unsatisfied.

Sublimation as Educational Aim

The fact, mentioned above, that the only good results from the present system of education come from the disguising of the unconscious wishes which strive for expression may be explained by saying that the only good derived from education is from sublimation. Education, from the side of the learner, is a form of sublimation. But sublimation is achieved not only in education. Indeed, it is achieved less through formal education, that is, by fewer persons than succeed in other ways in sublimating their unconscious wishes. And *the one aim of formal education ought to be sublimation.* I have stated this before in saying that the pupil should be taught to transfer his mental activity from the world of phantasy in which he was born to the world of reality into which he sometimes never is born. That is otherwise expressed by saying that the unconscious wish which in home education gets repressed before the child is old enough to go to school should first be recognized by educators, who never have recognized it, and then employed in sublimated forms, a thing that *has never yet been consciously done.* It could not, of course, be consciously done, because the very existence of the unconscious as a craving for life, love and activity was unknown.

But knowing, as we do now, something of the existence, the nature and the mechanisms of the unconscious wish, we shall gradually begin to be able to get hold of it, and to sublimate those portions of it which should be sublimated and give the individual a scientific knowledge of those portions which should not be sublimated. This could not have been done before today, because only today have we learned of the existence of the unconscious wish, any more than telephones could have been invented before the existence and nature of electricity had been discovered. But we can begin tomorrow, at any rate, if not today, to use the energies of this unconscious wish in the complete education, in the true sense of "drawing out" of it by means of our gradually increasing knowledge of its nature and mechanisms.

Rapport vs. *Quiz*

I imagine that the schools of the future will be conducted on a plan radically different from that now followed. There will be no "quizzes" and no attitude on the part of the teacher which suggests criticism of the work of the pupils, but there will be greater personal relation of *rapport* between pupil and teacher than ever could be now under the question-and-answer quiz-régime.

There is nothing in the whole present educational system better designed to emphasize and accentuate the unconscious antagonism between pupil and teacher than the teacher's simply asking the pupil a question and sitting eagle-eyed for the opportunity of swooping down upon any flaw in the answer. This comminuting of knowledge (in the place of the magnifying of wisdom) has reached such a degree of absurdity that teachers are marked for their success in eliciting complete sentences as answers to questions, where the performance of the pupil should not be a single sentence but a sustained verbal expression of an intellectual point of view or a feeling.

The unconscious antagonism of the pupil against the teacher is aroused by the implication contained in the very act of expressing the relation of the teacher to the pupil as a question about a statement in a book. The question implies the inability of the pupil to answer it properly, else why should it be put? If it is not put for the purpose of making one pupil wretchedly miserable because he cannot answer it at all, in the hope that he will be stirred by emulation if perchance another pupil in his " class " should be able to answer it, it is put with the design of bringing out the defective elements in the pupil's information, which of course his unconscious is most unwilling to have brought out and exhibited before the eyes of all his classmates—sometimes as many as sixty or seventy in some of the public schools of larger cities. And the question-putting method's effect on the teacher's unconscious makes him as impossible on his side as the pupil soon becomes on his own. The implication in the case of the teacher is that he is in a position to put the question and to correct the answer. There seems nothing extraordinary in this? The net result for the teacher is to make him more and more, as the years go on, merely a censorious critic, unless he instinctively, as many do, tends in the direction of sympathy for and interest in his pupils.

The situation of being placed in a position where it is one's duty to kill error may have delighted the soul of some puritanic ancient schoolmaster, but the modern way will be to ignore error and encourage right expression. The only way rightly to give attention to errors is to analyse the causes of why they were committed, and in the schools of the future, if there are enough educational analysts, that may be done and the result may be both interesting and profitable.

There will be no quizzes nor any quizziform attitude on the part of the teacher. Questioning by the teacher has also another implication, which is that the teacher thinks it is impossible to get an expression of the pupil's individuality in any other way. It may be physically impossible for the teacher to get that expression through questions because of the large numbers of pupils, but I am sure that it is impossible as a matter of mental mechanism to get any expression, not to say information, by means of the question form of attack by the teacher. As for questions in general one knows, even children know, that a sincere question is asked only for the purpose of getting *information* which the questioner has not. And when it comes to playing or making believe that the teacher *wants* to know the " answers " to the questions which he propounds, any child can play at that game, if it so desires, out of school, when it plays school, and there is little sense in making this double pretence in a school where real things ought to be. The child has to pretend that the teacher needs to be told things, and the teacher has to pretend that he is very anxious to learn. On the other hand, children are very much interested, of course, to acquire bits of information which the teacher has not. From this point of view the only interesting teacher is the vulnerable one, the one in whose knowledge, since it is a matter of knowledge concerning things which are in themselves hopelessly uninteresting, holes can be poked. The rare teacher who is absolutely master of his subject is naturally unavailable for this kind of entertainment. One cannot corner him

or find a weak spot in him any more than in a wall of
rock. His mental façade has been set in mortar
years ago, and is unsusceptible to any changing by any
efforts that a pupil could bring to bear on him. If
nothing can be done with him, what earthly interest
has he?

It is idle to think that children are interested in subjects in the curriculum as such. They are mildly interested in the teachers for a few hours or minutes until
they have been classified as cross, pleasant, good (efficient) or bad (inefficient), and then the interest returns
to the perennial one—interest in each other and the effects they can produce on each other. Very clever children can produce effects on other children by learning
the lessons with ease, reciting them with fluency and
asking the teacher sly questions, all of which place such
a child in the limelight of the classroom stage, in which
the other children, not the teacher, are the audience.
The other children, not being able to shine in this artificial activity, are forced either to give up the idea of
effecting any change on their environment, or to devote
their energies, whose legitimate object is the effecting
of such a change, to producing that effect on their companions. Hence spit-balls.

It was stated at the beginning of this section that
the main purpose of education is the causing of unconscious thought by conscious action. If this is so,
what is the effect of the conscious actions which take place
in such large numbers in the schoolroom upon the unconscious thoughts of the scholars? Nobody has ever
taken the trouble to consider that point except remotely
in the general statement that bad lessons and bad conduct

are a bad example for the pupil; therefore good conduct should be insisted on by the teacher.

The question of the invisible effect boys and girls produce on each other by being in a schoolroom together has been answered both ways by separating them and by coeducating them. But very few, even educators, know even instinctively what harm the conscious actions of the boys can do to the unconscious thoughts of the girls and vice versa, or what good. And they do not know the nature of the damage caused by bringing up girls in female academies and sending boys away to boys' " prep " schools.

Another Aim

The causing of unconscious thought by means of conscious acts as a purpose of education will not be agreed to by all pedagogues, because there is no accurate way of measuring the effect on the unconscious thought caused by the conscious action; if we cannot see the effect, how can we measure it? how know that what we do has any, or the right, effect? This is very unsatisfactory, because in our present day question and answer, lecture and reading and advanced seminar style of education, one can get immediate measurements or estimates of the conscious effect produced by conscious action. We note them down, in fact, proportioned on a scale of 100, and mail these notes frequently to parents. We ask the pupil and find out immediately just what he knows and how much effect we have had on his conscious mental activity by our conscious actions, and if the effect has not been sufficient we increase the cause. This would seem to express the blind way in which present systems work.

As a matter of fact there is absolutely no sure standard by which the unconscious thought-effect, derived from conscious activity, can possibly be numerically measured. The effect caused in the unconscious by conscious activity can, however, now be traced, and it will not be long before it can be more accurately known than the conscious. It is, of course, estimated by indirect methods, but these are more sure than the direct methods of question and answer, laboratory note book and thesis, which are used to estimate the conscious progress of the student.

It is a well-known fact that the amount of conscious mental activity necessary to graduate from any school or college is comparatively small, and is easily accomplished by some persons, who are free from the inhibitions so common to all others, in half to three-quarters of the time usually taken. The reason why the average student spends four years in doing the high-school work, and from four to six years in doing the college work, is that he is influenced by tradition and other suggestions to believe that the work is hard and must take so long. Another reason is that there is in both secondary and higher educational methods an inordinate amount of time wasted, during which the pupil or student is actually retarded so that the slowest may keep up with him. There is no reason why all boys and girls of a certain grade of maturity should not do all the preparation for college in one year instead of four, if they were willing to do it, and if at the same time they were not actually prevented by the present methods of recitations in large classes from going ahead as fast as they can. The actual procedure in a so-called recitation is a method of the most dreary slowness compared with the vivacity with which the individuals composing the class attack problems no less intellectual, when they understand the importance and vitality of the subjects for their own lives.

Function of the Teacher of the Future

So that the duty of the teacher of the future will be to prepare the disposition of the pupil for the acquirement of knowledge and not to give instructon itself. It would appear, if at the present time such a practice were carried on, that the teacher was not minding his business, for he would not immediately begin talking to his pupils about the lesson but would take them one at a time, and would at once begin to listen to a fellow-human talk about himself. Only in this way, by patient listening, can the teacher know a student. It has long been known that *Magister Johannem Latinum docet* implies that the teacher knows Latin if he is to teach Latin, and furthermore that he knows John. Up to date his knowledge of John has been a knowledge only of John's exterior superficial consciousness. In the schools of the future " magister " will be required to know about John's unconscious, to have a knowledge both of its nature and the means of inferring it from his acts, words and other expressions.

In order to get this knowledge he will have to learn from John more than he will ever be able to teach him, although the results of his knowledge of John's unconscious will be communicated to John and will be of far greater use to him than any other knowledge he now gains in school or college.

So that in the place of recitations of large classes in

which very little of human relation emerges, except petty rivalry, teasing and other forms of unconscious manifestations, there will be only a continual conference in private between the teacher and the pupils one at a time. The curriculum of cultural and other studies now covered can be increased in amplitude almost *ad infinitum,* if that still seems advisable, and the pupil will go from the teacher's study or conference room to the laboratory, the library, the gymnasium or the workshops and work with complete devotion, as soon as he understands the vitality of social relations.   To the teacher especially equipped to teach expression in English he will go with an essay or extemporary speech, a problem or a series of questions, all suggested by his own thinking and working on the problems of life as he sees it.

This will not necessarily do away with team work in learning.   One of the great advantages will be that all school work will be done in school, and none of it in the interruptions of desultory home life, a condition which makes it at present so very hard for school children to do any work at home.   The value of most children's home work is almost *nil.*   There will be discussions of the points which come up in the literature read both in English and in foreign languages, and there will be conversational meetings for the foreign language students. Pupils will be encouraged to study together where such combined methods do not tend to strengthen the stronger of the two and weaken the weaker, as is now so frequently the case.

Attention will be given, in a way impossible now in schools, to the development of the mental and moral as well as of the physical factors in the individual, and a development of them in a reasonable and scientific proportion. If athletics are good for some, they are good for all, and there will be provision made for all to share in them; but if it is found that they are unnecessary for all, as may very well be the case, it will not be recommended for all. In any case there will be an opportunity, not now afforded, for the teacher to be in a position to know in detail of the needs of the individual as indicated by his now utterly unexplored unconscious, and put him in the way of satisfying those needs to a degree that is not now possible, and never has been possible, except in the rarest cases, such, for instance, as those of John Stuart Mill and Thomas De Quincey; and in cases like the latter, the element which led to his taking opium can be detected and the unconscious wish impelling him to that course can be directed, in the newer education, to other and socially more available aims.

Religion and Sex

The great questions of religion and sex, so closely related in the history of the individual as well as in that of the race, will be answered both in language so scientific that it will obviate the objections by which they are now practically ruled out of the schools except where they exist in a vestigial, rudimentary and completely devitalized condition, although they are questions which occupy the unconscious mentality of all persons all the time. The erroneous solutions of the problems connected with religion and sex are responsible for a large part of the crime, disease and even war itself—that running amuck of the unconscious wish.

Alongside of these much more weighty questions of religion and sex, both of which are so intimately connected with the primordial craving of the ego, the actual accomplishment of what are now such burdensome tasks for pupil and student will seem as nothing. It is a fact that a desire to satisfy sexual and religious curiosity, if not gratified in a natural and wholesome manner, may be the cause of much mental and moral confusion in later life. It is also a fact that these two fields of human curiosity are opened very early in life, and that they are explored without proper guidance, both because well-informed guides are few and far between, and because those who attempt to instruct young people in these two subjects are necessarily full of error coming from an ignorance of the unconscious and of psychical mechanisms generally.

It has been proved again and again that children who receive warped views of the sexual relations in the narrow sense of genital sexuality, which they do at a surprisingly early age, receive therein a stamp which gives a perverted form to every subsequent impression, just as a mirror once broken into a dozen pieces will always thereafter reflect light at a dozen different angles, and as a concrete sidewalk trodden when soft by a dog will always retain the footprints. The removal of these false or warped impressions will be effected when the soul is plastic, in the days even before adolescence, with greater ease and surety than it possibly could be later in life. Medical psychology of the analytic type is concerned chiefly in the remoulding of these early fortuitous and ill-balanced patterns in persons who have, because of the pressure of circumstances, become neurotics. The cause of the neu-

rosis is always found to be a warping of the soul at a
very early day, much as if exposed too early to the flames
of love. The sensibilities of such people may be likened,
too, to the warped condition of the lens of the eye which
produces astigmatism, or to the paralysing of the muscles
of   accommodation   which   produces   near-sightedness.
Such people's physical vision is always defective and must
be corrected with artificial lenses. The spiritual vision
of the neurotic, the satisfaction of whose early sexual
curiosity has not been complete, leaving him to make erroneous reasonings of his own about the things most
personal and intimate to him, is similarly warped, and
all his life, unless he has the fortune to fall into the hands
of an experienced medical psychologist, he sees the realities of life in a very much distorted form, due to the
warping of his spiritual lens. The proper treatment can
either supply him with an artificial one or straighten out
his own.

And so the ordinary subjects of the curriculum will in
the schools of the future retire in importance before the
one great question of the sanitation of the sexual impluses
in both the broad and the narrow sense. In speaking
of sexuality in the narrow sense I mean of course the
specifically genital sexuality which comes into existence at
puberty. Definite information which is now not possessed
by the majority of married couples on this point will undoubtedly have to be given first in the schools, by men
teachers to boys and to girls by married women teachers.
It will have to be given first in the schools because it is impossible to instruct the mothers and fathers of children
how to tell them the real facts of sex, both because they
do not know these facts and because there is an uncon-

scious cause why it is more difficult for parents to talk to their own children about such matters. Later, when several generations of children, clear-eyed in their view of reproductive and productive creation and the relations between them, have had children of their own, it may be possible for the schools to leave the matter in the hands of parents. At present, however, it is amply manifest that parents are generally incompetent to handle the matter themselves. No teacher who knows fails to see in almost all the adolescent children under his care the signs of unsatisfied sexual curiosity in their actions and in their attitude toward intellectual matters.

Sexuality in a Broad Sense

Sexuality in the broad sense, however, has to be considered in every action which the individual performs, and the manner in which he relates the broadly sexual to the specifically genital sexual is of the greatest importance to him in his entire philosophy of life. The sexual questions, both in the broad and in the narrow sense, are pondered by each boy and girl, each man and woman, according to their nature and environment and their experience. There is no human being who is not either a man or a woman or destined to become one, and the problems of sex *are* faced by each and every one of us in his or her own way. Everyone has a philosophy of life based on his relation to the life which he bears and which it is his duty to transmit. Upon the proper solution of these problems depend his or her health and happiness. They form the core of existence and the root of all good and evil. Mankind has with consistent errancy averted its gaze from the essential to the non-essential under the impression that the narrowly sexual would take care of itself if only the externals were carefully looked after. In many cases, therefore, it has sedulously watered a plant at whose root was a cutworm which they could and should but would not see.

Part of this aversion to look sexuality squarely in the eye comes from an infantile attitude toward the parent. It comes about in two ways first because of a positive prohibition on the father's or mother's part. They tell the child not to think of such subjects. A little girl is made the object of one of the very common sexual investigations carried on by children in their unwatched hours sometimes before their fifth year. In instinctive terror she runs home to her mother and begins to tell her the circumstances. Her mother hushes her up with " Awful! " and " Unspeakable! " or words to that effect. The little girl thinks that some terrible calamity has befallen her, and that probably she is disgraced for life. She hangs her head for months and is told by her mother, who is ignorant of the child mind, to stand up straight and act better, all of which confirms the poor child's suspicions that she has done something which has made it impossible for her ever to hold up her head properly. She later forgets all about it, voluntarily represses it from her consciousness because it is painful to her, this innocent childish incident which, if explained to her by a sympathetic and intelligent mother, would never have so depressed her for so long a time. Eventually she succeeds in forgetting it, but the impression it made upon her, together with her mother's attitude toward it, has left an imprint on her psyche which makes impossible for her the clear gaze at reality which ought to be the right of every human. Out of a really trivial episode the mother made an intolerably terrible experience for the blameless child and filled her mind with a wholly unjust sense of guilt which spoiled her forever for seeing things as they really are. This child is spiritually in much the same condition as the babies who, through carelessness or ignorance on the part of the physician, are made blind at birth, or cripples, and ever after are unable to see or walk as the case may be. Such a permanent twist is given very frequently in the earliest childhood, and is manifested sometimes forty or fifty years later.

The Mother-Infant Attitude

Now if this twist is existent in a large number of people, if they have, we shall not call it a weakness but a twist or warp which is going to run the wrong way of the tension some day just because the grain of the wood, so to speak, crosses the oar at the oarlock; if we never know what sort of an abyss we may be walking near, we are in a condition which is not so good and advantageous and up-to-date as that condition would be where we knew just how we stood. For if we knew how we stood, we should be in a position to take steps in the right direction. Not knowing how we stand is very much like being satisfied to leave everything to fate. If we are resigned to leave everything to fate, which is constituted for most of us by external reality, we are like children who are satisfied to take everything they get from the mother and have not the ideas to look for or require more. It is only very young children who are thus content, in fact only infants. So the attitude toward the world which accepts the world as fate is an excessively infantile attitude. It is only through an active pursuit in the external world after things which are suggested by internal mental activities, that we leave the Fate Attitude or the Mother-Infant Attitude. If, in other words, we are convinced, as I believe every thinking person is, that there is any knowledge attainable by us, which will give us more power over external reality, we show immediately our adult attitude in making every effort to attain that knowledge.

The knowledge of the unconscious and of its mechanisms is a knowledge which gives power not only over the external world but the mental, and gives power over it solely because of the added knowledge which it gives us of ourselves, our nature, our abilities, our loves, our hates, likes, dislikes, mannerisms and modes of thought.

Methods More Elastic

With the change of front on the part of the teacher made possible by the newer standpoint, a change of front from the group to the individual, will come a very great difference in the rate at which the subject-matter is covered. It will be possible if not probable that a student will devote more time consecutively to a given subject. It is characteristic of children to act with great enthusiasm and concentration, when once their interests are aroused. A student of sixteen just said to me, " I get waked up after about an hour," meaning that she became thoroughly interested and eager to go on. I replied that frequently I got waked up myself, after an hour or two, to a state of activity which seemed impossible at the beginning of any bit of work.

The ringing of a bell in a recitation room of the twentieth century breaks off a great deal of unconscious activity which, being slow in getting up a momentum, is in some natures jarred by a sudden coming to a standstill or a shunting off on another track. I feel sure that in the schools of the future a subject will be studied by a student intensively, and naturally so, until a point is reached where a solid satisfaction is experienced by the student over a good-sized job done completely. This may take a whole day or several days. I see no reason why, for instance, Latin should not be studied in high school until a year's work is finished, say in ten weeks, and an examination taken. Then the subject could be temporarily dropped in favor of some other. In this way a student might finish off first and get credit for subjects that were easier for him and leave the harder ones for the time of his greater maturity. This is the more reasonable as there is so very great a change in the mental maturity of pupils between the ages of thirteen and seventeen.

This elastic plan would allow some girls, for instance, who on entering high school are totally unfit for mathematics to postpone them until their fourth year. This is the year in which a great many pass successfully the work of the first year in mathematics, which however they have been taking term after term and failing in. They could, indeed, omit the study of mathematics entirely, if, and only if, an analysis of the pupil should indicate that she was a case of utter inability to master mathematics. This would not often be the case, because the careful analysis by the teacher would reveal and remove the causes lying in the unconscious of the pupil, causes which make the mathematics difficult. It would then be not difficult, but very easy.

It has been found that young people's interest in or distaste for a given subject is often conditioned not by any innate quality of their mental constitution but by their attitude toward it, which has been determined for them by some early impression made upon them by a parent or brother or sister. In the case of one boy on record it was not any incapacity of his own which rendered his learning of scientific subjects almost impossible, but it was the fact that his father had excelled in that branch, and had made very exacting requirements upon the boy to do very well in that subject, and was inept enough to express disappointment in, and resentment at, the boy for not showing an aptitude for them at once. How many special teachers know whether or not the signal failures of a pupil to do well in their subjects are caused by some home influence such as this? No discredit to them, to be sure, for not knowing, for not only do they lack the instrumentality to ascertain but they also have not at present the time to find out. Just as the difficulty of the scientific subjects was removed for the boy above mentioned when he was helped to understand why he could not do well in that subject, so in the future will any such difficulty be removed by an understanding given him by his adviser, tracing the cause of this difficulty. A difficulty of this nature is almost invariably the result of an inhibition on the part of the boy or girl caused by some fancied relation of that subject to their father or mother. It is a relation, too, that is generally not consciously known

to the pupil, so how could the teacher, not knowing anything of the unconscious, or the pupil, who also does not
know, ever find out and illuminate this relation?

Many times in the present system of education a pupil
fails in a subject, drops it and takes up another in place
of it because he fancies the other will be " easier." How
does he know that French is easier than Latin? Is it
or is it not? He does not know. He thinks it is, and
frequently he thinks it is, because his mother or father
want him to study Latin. If the parent advises Latin,
the unconscious antagonism between parent and child
(which exists everywhere and involves no blame to either
parent or child, because neither knows of its existence)
makes some other language take on a much greater
attractiveness, partly because, not being the parent's
choice, it thereby immediately can be exclusively the
child's choice. This conflict is partly conscious, partly
unconscious, in varying degrees in different cases. If the
subject is chosen exclusively by the child, he is of course
consciously or unconsciously on his own mettle to do
well in it, and all the more so if there is some opposition
on the part of the parent.

Summary

The unconscious unwillingness of pupils to do school
work is caused by the early impressions received from
their parents, whose influence, due to pardonable ignorance, is very bad for the later welfare of their children.
The parent has the great responsibility of creating the
mind of the child, a process which must be maintained
for at least five years after birth. The worst influence

exerted by the parent is a failure to satisfy the child's inevitable sex curiosity. The effects of a perverted handling of this topic or a refusal to treat it properly gives a twist to the child's understanding not only of the most fundamental human relations but also of the things of the world apparently most remote from the sexual. The difference between directed and undirected thinking, showing the unconscious wish as a tension, brings out the fact that all humans have a continuous wish or tension toward creation, either reproductive or productive. The occurrence of ideas to the mind is discussed and the true meaning of thoughtless acts, which shows both teacher and parent a more scientific attitude with regard to attaching blame to children. The question of the policy of trying to strengthen what parents and teachers consider the weak points of the child is discussed from the point of view of organ inferiority. The unfortunate trend in academic education to date has been to turn the child away from reality. Possible reality in the child's school life is comparatively small, although the advantages of an early acquaintance with it would be invaluable. The school in the distant future may be the homes of the people. At present, however, all the teacher can do is to reproduce in the atmosphere created by him in the schoolroom as much as possible of the quality of reality. An example is given of how a high-school teacher succeeded in reproducing in his classroom some of the extra-mural social environment which is not found in many schools.

Some of the specific aims of education from the point of view of psychoanalysis are given: to alter the psychical environment, to amplify consciousness, to remove unconscious fear, to sublimate the unconscious desires. The function of the teacher of the future will not be to ask questions, but to elicit the mental activity of the child, and only incidentally to straighten out misconceptions with regard to sex. The attitude of the person knowing something about the unconscious and not striving to know more is regarded as the Fate or Mother-Infant attitude. A greater elasticity will be available in the school of the future, whereby a pupil will be enabled to take up subjects more in accordance with their suitability to his stage of mental development. In brief, the aims of education including both academic education and that outside of schools, are first to separate the child from himself, in such way that he can exert his efforts primarily to effect a change upon the world of external reality, which is indeed the best way in which to effect a change upon himself; to transmute physical energy into psychical energy, which is much more mobile and productive, a phase of which constitutes sublimation; to unite consciousness and the unconscious, thereby producing the most vigorous personality, making everything he does most intensely personal. The net result of all these aims will be the uniting of the child again with reality, but in a different sense from that in which he was united with reality at birth. It is pointed out in various places how the conscious education fails to unite the parts of the individual personality.

CHAPTER VII

RESISTANCE AND TRANSFERENCE

THE attitude of children toward their school work is an index both of conscious and of unconscious wishes. Some children are unduly downcast by failure to do passing work, and some are unduly unmoved by their failures. Some have enough density of psychical epidermis, so to speak, instinctively to make due allowance for the unconscious conflicts in the teacher's own personality, and to avoid being disturbed by what the teacher says, and also to take advantage of the teacher's unconscious conflicts. In the latter case the pupil takes a pleasure in making the teacher unhappy, just as he naturally takes pleasure in playing on the emotions of his elders at home and of the chance acquaintances of the street. The street person, however, he treats with a certain amount of wariness because the unknown may contain unpleasant surprises in the way of powerful opposition or control. At home he has the advantage of knowing the peculiarities of his relatives, and he can pull the same old strings repeatedly with great success, while in school he has the advantage of being shielded by numbers, and of being able to act in a concerted attack upon the enemy representative of authority. This is the normal unconscious attitude of the not over-sadistic healthy individual, and is determined by his unconscious wishes.

The child, on the other hand, who takes school too

seriously, who spends many hours on the preparation of his lessons, even if they *are* hard, is one who has not learned the chief or at least one of the chief lessons which one learns at the present-day school—namely, the art of discounting the apparent requirements of the environment. For teachers are constantly setting tasks which cannot be well performed by the majority of pupils, working as they do against the great resistances which are inevitable in all school work. These resistances are unknown even to the children themselves. The children think they want to learn and will honestly say that they want to learn, but as a matter of pure " brass tacks " nobody wants to learn *from another person,* even from a professional teacher. The greater the authority with which the teacher is invested, the greater will be the unconscious resistance, naturally and normally, against it. And as the authority with which the teacher is upholstered increases his magnitude in his own eyes, and gives a profound satisfaction to one of his strongest, but still unconscious, wishes, his acts in the classroom inevitably tend toward the assertion of authority and to the idea that his aim is to impress upon the pupil from without a body of information which will increase his (the pupil's) efficiency ultimately and give him power and authority. If the teacher is not keenly aware that he is feeding on *unconscious* desire in making the pupils do what he thinks they should, he runs the very great risk of giving too great an emphasis to the authoritative element in his teaching.

Authoritative Attitude of Teachers

Another very great incentive to the teacher to become authoritative is due to the fact that, in a sphere in which the pupils are not particularly interested, their own unconscious makes them see many difficulties and they crave guidance and assistance. This may seem to contradict the statement that they instinctively resist authority, but it is really no contradiction. For the authority which they resist is the one that requires them to attend to subjects which do not primarily appeal to their instincts. The very existence of a curriculum and a time-table and a programme and the ringing of bells, which always interrupt when interest is finally aroused, the very nature of requirement itself is one that creates unconscious resistance which is shown in tardiness, in absence, both physical manifestations, and also in inattention, which is the psychical manifestation of unconscious resistance.

One Result of Resistance

A condition which results from this unconscious resistance is that it is practically impossible to tell anybody anything, chiefly for the reason that the act of telling implies a superiority on the part of the teller, which has to be admitted by the listener, and this the listener's unconscious is quite unable to admit. The only way in which a concrete result can be obtained—a result in which there is any dynamic factor having an influence on the actions of the person here called listener—is the indirect method of turning the listener himself into a teller, a process which seems completely to reverse the main principles of education as they are generally practised. The teacher then ostensibly becomes the learner and the pupil gives information.

The True Question

The art of teaching, then, consists in following the Socratic " maieutic " method of developing or " delivering " the thoughts, and by means of them the actions, of the pupil, who all along is to be assured that he is imparting information * which the teacher is sincerely desirous of knowing. And it does not take so great a transformation, after all, on the part of the teacher, to make him feel that, by listening to the conscious thoughts of the pupil, he can soon gain a leverage on the pupil's unconscious thoughts, after he has discovered what they are by a survey of their manifestations in conscious thought and action. In this way he can influence the pupil without the pupil's knowing it, an influence which we know to be all the more potent the less aware of it the pupil is.

---

* I do not refer to information about history or English literature or French or Spanish or mathematics. I do not hesitate to assert the insincerity of the statement " Now I want to know " or " I want you to tell me about " this or that topic in the school curriculum is an insincerity which is always immediately sensed by the pupil, and absolutely vitiates any educational value that this form of encounter between teacher and pupil is supposed to have. But in saying that the teacher is to receive information from the pupil, I mean information about the pupil's own self, the conscious elements of which will to the skilful teacher inevitably reveal the existence and form of the unconscious elements of which the pupil himself has not the remotest knowledge. In this way school and college education will take a step in the direction of real penetrating analysis. It cannot become a thorough analysis, for the reason that there will not be time enough for it, but it will, if it goes any distance at all, on that line, be an infinite advance over anything that is being done today in schools. One step is infinitely greater than no step at all.

An important corollary of this principle that it is impossible to tell anybody anything (except in the case where so simple and impersonal a question is asked as " What time is it? " or " What was the thermometer at three this afternoon? ") is in the evident futility of the teacher doing much talking, an unfortunate practice which is very prevalent in schools. The unconscious of the child is soothed, by the hypnotic monotony of the teacher's voice, into an inattentive and dreamy state most conducive to pure undirected thinking or phantasying. The unconscious of the teacher is enormously gratified by the sense of power which is given him by his fluent speech evidencing his mastery of his " subject." In the schools of the future the subject will have to be changed for the *ob*ject, the child. Then the child will become fluent and from observation of the teacher may himself learn when to hold his own tongue.

One reason why the simple question as to matter of fact, e.g. concerning the actual time, gives the opportunity to tell a person something is that the question contains comparatively much, and the answer contains comparatively little, of the personal element—the unconscious element, the wish element. When I want to know the time, I really do not care who tells me, provided I get reasonably correct information from a person reasonably willing to give it. The amount of wish-energy put forth and satisfied by the person who has the watch or can see the clock, is almost infinitesimal under ordinary conditions. A glance and a couple of words and *his* performance is complete, except if he be infantile—either a child or a child-minded adult. If he is a small boy with his first watch, he may develop a large amount of wish-energy in connection with his answer, or if it is a girl who has any interest in our actions. But ordinarily this piece of human relationship is marked by a large amount of wish-energy in the one person and a very small amount in the other.

I take this to be a type of the relation which should exist between teacher and pupil. In it the person asking the time represents the pupil and the owner of the time-piece the teacher. But I observe that the relation between pupil and teacher is generally quite the reverse. The teacher, and particularly one who is " full of his subject," will talk by the hour, putting his material year by year into a more highly organized form and becoming a better and better expositor or " putter-forth." In all of this progress in his own intellectual development he does not in the least degree reach his students better. He does nothing but increase his own fluency, and in any grade of education below the university, increase the breadth of his own knowledge.

The True Answer

Education on the contrary should be more a matter of extraction from the pupil than exposition by the teacher. The pupil must himself acquire the knowledge. Knowledge exposed by the teacher is but knowledge, and, as we all know only too well, extensively unrelated to the wish-energy of the pupil. Knowledge acquired by the pupil's efforts is wisdom, but no knowledge is acquired from a source too energetic. One cannot get a drink from a high-pressure fire hose, no matter how thirsty one is.

A true teacher therefore is necessarily one who can give the brief and impersonal answer of the person telling the time, and freed entirely from any wish-energy applied directly to the act of imparting information. But so insidiously does the teacher's unconscious control his actions that he is constantly, and in ignorance of the true state of affairs, satisfying, before the audience of his classroom, the desire for self-exploitation, a very natural one to be sure, and characterizing all persons but most profitable to society only in professional entertainers.

If the ideal education is to consist of a drawing out of the powers of the child with the aim of having him devote those energies to effecting a change, not in himself, but in the external world, the question arises of the means and the method for developing in the child the desire to work upon that portion of the external world chosen by the framers of the curriculum. For children do not instinctively give up the undirected thinking (day-dreaming or phantasying) which is the easy, because internal, manner of satisfying their unconscious wishes, and substitute for it the mode of thinking directed toward the world of reality, which is a difficult mode because it requires an effort physically expended upon the reality of the world external to himself.

This applies most closely, of course, to the abstract and so-called cultural subjects in the curriculum. If we are to have the student really satisfying a real desire in getting an education, that desire must be satisfied not only at the end of a part of it as when he receives a school diploma or a college or university degree, but must be satisfied moment by moment during the progress of his work. Every bit of information he gets from the teacher must be gotten for the purpose of satisfying a bit of desire, and we know how infrequently that is the case in the schools of the present, where the teacher, called also instructor (or he that piles upon), is largely a task-master or slave driver, necessarily on account of the demands of the syllabus.

It is absolutely necessary that the information must be, for its best effect upon the soul of the student, gotten in the heat of desire, for only then is it fused so that it becomes a vital part of his unconscious mentality. There is no doubt that every impression made upon any sentient being is retained forever. All the lessons and tasks of school, all the lectures and essays of college are permanently stored in the unconscious, but they have never been vitalized because they were passively received, and not actively acquired. This is clear when we reflect that the rhythm of tension and relaxation, which constitutes the actual dynamics of psychical life, is the fundamental mechanism by which the psyche develops, exactly as metabolism is a rhythm of anabolism and catabolism in animal physiology.

Constant Tension and Relaxation

The unconscious tensions or wishes of the human individual are from minute to minute relaxed and tensed. This rhythm of tension or wish and relaxation or gratification goes on from moment to moment in the mental (as well as in the physical) life of each one of us. It is going on with the regularity, if not with the rapidity, of the heart beat, in every child in every classroom. In those students who get the most out of their school educa-

tion the desire and its gratification are centred in the subject-matter of the course they are pursuing or else in the
attitude of themselves to their teachers or in that of their
teachers to them.   Such students, dubbed grinds by
others, are not always the best men and women.   Very
frequently they are a great disappointment after they
have graduated, and can succeed in life only as per-
petuators of the same system of education in which they
were brought up.   They become teachers themselves
(who ever heard of a successful teacher who felt con-
tempt for the subject he was teaching?) and they strive
to put their pupils through the same pattern which
stamped themselves.   Having been themselves stencilled,
they naturally think everybody else ought to be stencilled,
and with the same shapes.

But there are others whose instincts or unconscious
wishes cannot be satisfied with the material which is offered them in the schools.   Why they cannot remains a
problem yet to be discussed.   With book geography, with
spelling, with English compositions, Latin, algebra and
what not, they cannot ally their unconscious wishes.
Their conscious wishes they do so affiliate with the educational topics selected for them by their elders, and they
pretend to a desire for book learning partly because of
the social status given to it.

But during every minute of their existence in any educational institution, just as much as when they are out
of it, all students are forming and satisfying desires, unconscious ones mainly.   And the rhythm of tension and
relaxation, of desire and gratification, goes on constantly.
It expresses the most vital factor in the life of the individual.   Those who say (and show) that they have no

conscious desires, the listless ones, are the ones whose desires are all unconscious, either repressed or not yet manifested. All people however constantly have desire, and whether it is conscious or unconscious depends largely upon their environment. If their surroundings have been such as to repress their instinctive desires that have emerged from time to time (Johnny mustn't *do THAT!*) and they have not been able to substitute acceptable desires and gratifications for the prohibited ones, then the desires are mostly unconscious and the individuals so hampered are more or less in the condition of manacled slaves, or imprisoned felons. What is the history of the vital rhythm of desire and satisfaction, of wish and fulfilment in these persons?

Let it be remembered that as a wish is actually a material physical tension in muscles of the living human body and as only the relaxation of the tension is the satisfaction of that wish, it is a physical impossibility that any wish should remain ungratified. In other words *every human desire* is thus *always being fulfilled* in one way or another. There is no tension which during life is not relaxed, to make way for another tension, just as there is no life consisting of pure inactivity or absolute relaxation. Even in a hibernating animal, changes take place which are manifested on his reappearance in the spring. The absolutely relaxed is actually dead.

If every human wish is fulfilled in some way, it is quite evident that if it is not consciously fulfilled it must be unconsciously. The unconscious of each and every individual is an unlimited store of material for wish fulfilment. The very act of relaxation, even that coming through fatigue, is a fulfilment of a wish in so far as it is the relaxation of a tension. And as the tensions will relax, even though the intended gratification is not actually secured, we find ourselves, possessed as we are with a faculty of mental reproduction of sensations, deriving our satisfactions from ideal, imaginary internal sources, instead of the external ones which have disappointed us.

That is what takes place every day in every schoolroom. The unconscious wishes of the child, denied an actual external gratification, inevitably seek and find an internal one. That is what is going on before your eyes, Mr. and Miss Teacher and Mr. and Mrs. Parent, every day of your life. For the solution of the problem of what to do with and even how to get hold of the unconscious wishes of the student has not up to the present time had any light thrown on it. In fact, the problem as such has not been presented at all. Education has treated the student as a being all conscious and no part unconscious. In so doing it has disregarded the most essential point and its problems so far have been merely superficial and the solutions nugatory.

Teachers Commonly Ignorant of Wish Rhythm

This, then, is the real problem of education. If we are to educate, we must know what we have to educate. If we are ourselves going to effect a result on a part of external reality (our pupils), we have to know something about it. As educators we seem to have had the idea that we wanted a child's pale face to be red or green, and to have laid on thick coats of red paint or green, and to have wondered why they did not sink into and become a part of his tissue, not knowing that the only way to give him red cheeks is to let him exercise his own muscles. We thought his face was pale! Possibly the paleness was in our own vision. Healthy children, not aligned and rigidified by school furniture, are red-cheeked anyway. If we are to help Nature we must know something about her. If we wish, and think we have a right, to change human nature, we must know it as anatomists know the human body, as osteologists, as histologists, as cytologists. We must have a more accurate knowledge of psychical anatomy and histology. There is such a knowledge, the beginnings of which took place at the end of the nineteenth century and which is making great advances today.

As teachers we must learn and avail ourselves of the mechanisms of the unconscious mentality. We shall not feel the necessity of learning about them, if we do not know their existence, but, once our attention is called to them, we cannot fail to see them, as they are always there, functioning before our eyes. They have been visible but unseen forever, like any other obvious thing such as the air, whose chemical constituents are not an object of visual sensation and can never become so, but whose existence is a necessary postulate of chemical science, in explaining phenomena which are visible. Similarly we explain by things inaudible those which are audible, and in general we explain and understand the perceptible by means of things imperceptible. Thus do we explain conscious thought and act by means of the unconscious and its modes of functioning, which are, to be sure, somewhat different from the conscious, and have to be learned just as conscious processes can be learned (the various arts), but they are, although different, yet subject to the same natural laws as conscious mental processes.

If some knowledge is necessary for a physician to set a broken limb, surely as much knowledge as possible is advantageous for the teacher to set or reduce a broken disposition. In school children most broken dispositions are broken before they come to school and the teacher's duty, hitherto conceived to be but the dressing up of broken limbs in silks and laces, which only serve to disguise deformities, is really to strip off, at present to ignore, what uncouth sartorial integuments he finds on his pupils and pay sole attention to the reshaping of their badly deformed mental physique.

If as teachers we were required to know nothing except the nature of the veneer we attempt to apply, we should neither be interested in, nor know of the existence of, the bodies over which we plastered our thin films. But the moment we begin to believe that our concern is with the organism, whose color only, so to speak, we were formerly interested in, we become mental physicians instead of mental tailors.

Blindness of Humanity to Inner Wish Life

It will be admitted that humanity has been ostensibly more interested in the coverings of the body than in the body itself, and that just as it required a thousand years, more or less, for physicians as a profession to have any social position, so it will require some time for a teacher who knows as much about the mind as a medical man does about the body to gain repute for his knowledge and honor for his profession. There has always been as much disinclination on the part of humanity in general to have the real nature of its soul examined as there has been reluctance on the part of individual humans to have their bodies investigated. There is so-called modesty and fear in both cases. Knowledge, and particularly self-knowledge, has been too terrible for most minds. Many persons would be as unwilling to look into their own minds as into their own brain fissures, and possibly for the majority of people either of these is quite unnecessary. But for the teacher, who is to act in some sort analogously to the physician, a knowledge of, and an ability to see the undraped workings of the mind is a necessity.

That the educator has not had this intimate knowledge has not been his fault, for until lately nobody has had it. Until the time of the psychology of the unconscious wish, originated by Sigmund Freud and the different schools which have already developed in more or less divergent lines from his teachings, the unconscious, as a medium over which some control could be exercised by conscious effort, had been neither recognized nor investigated. It is Freud's use of his knowledge of the unconscious in the cure of hysteria and some other nervous diseases which has been extended from abnormal to normal psychology and has given a point of view from which much more can be learned of the human psyche than ever before.

Now we are beginning to have this vast and unexplored mental hinterland (to use H. G. Wells' expression) provisionally charted, we are able to look forward to a time when its inconceivably vast treasures will be available for more and more persons. Educators should be among the first to explore this hinterland as the physiographical conditions of it so constantly affect the climate of the coastal consciousness. Furthermore, human enter-

prise is gradually more and more opening up this hinterland of the mind, whose geological strata have been laid
down during the eons of time during which consciousness
has evolved out of inanimate matter.

Every teacher is aware, while facing a roomful of
lively children, that he is "up against" a collection of
wills, but now the knowledge comes that these variegated
volitions are not merely conscious purposes, but are unconscious wishes and that all of them are being fulfilled
continuously in his very presence.   There are no disap-
pointments and frustrations except the conscious ones.
Every unconscious wish struggles up toward the surface
of consciousness, and if repressed or inhibited, as most
of them are, by the teacher, they are immediately satisfied in the unconscious either by a perceptible movement
or by a thought.   The substitute satisfaction is always
taken in place of the one originally intended.   We desire
to breathe air.   If we are put in situations where we
breathe gas or chloroform or ether or water, breathing
movements go on just the same as long as the organism
lives.   The satisfaction of the unconscious wish is just
as instinctive and inevitable as that.

The marks made with knives and pencils on school
furniture or walls, the drawings and irrelevant words on
the pages of school-books, the dog's-ears, the blots, the
numerous traces of activity misdirected are all evidences
of the substitute satisfactions of the unconscious wishes
working through the conscious ones.   The uneasiness, the
antagonism, the slamming of books and occasional dropping of things on the floor, the surreptitious eating of
a bite of lunch and the chewing of gum are all attempts of
the unconscious to gain its own satisfaction in spite of the

restrictions put upon it by consciousness. The conscious wrangling of pupils with each other, and, where possible, with the teacher, are manifestations of the unconscious wish, sometimes a wish to exhibit, sometimes a generic wish for power. The attitude of mild or severe dislike of lessons or the apparent indifference, all these more undesirable expressions are expressions of the same unconscious.

There are desirable ones too. Every cheerful compliance on the part of the learner with the suggestions of the director of the learning, every thoughtful act of service done by the pupil for the teacher or the school is quite as much prompted by the unconscious as are the bad ones. I do not wish to give the unconscious an unduly black eye. By virtue of its enormous and unfailing power it can suggest and carry out really magnificent deeds, when at the same time its love of exhibition and mastery can be satisfied in doing them. The quickness with which the most unruly boys will rise to fine action in an emergency, the alacrity with which a nation goes to war, show the unconscious and the conscious life working together.

The actions of young people are more impulsive than those of older people because, as the older psychology would say, they are more instinctive and less reasoned. The newer psychology finds that instinct is the expression of the unconscious wishes and that they may sometimes in one action be at variance with reason and at other times in other actions coincide with reason. But this coincidence is rarer in youth than in later life and the actions of the young are therefore more " scatter-brained " and have less congruence with a social system than those of persons who have spent half a century or so in repressing, and finding, by the trial and error method, substitute satisfactions.

Unconscious Wishes Expressed in Idle Questions

Other examples of the unconscious wish fulfilment that is taking place every minute of every hour in the schoolroom are the foolish or perverse questions which are continually asked. I do not refer specially to the oft-repeated question: "What was *I* doing?", although the form of it shows the unconscious unwillingness on the part of the pupil to judge his own acts according to the conventional standards of the school. I refer here not to the questions which are asked about what page of the book the lesson is, or another kind of question which shows not a real difficulty and a desire to overcome it, a variety of question which is asked not in the recitation time but at the end of the school day or in a study period. I refer to a kind of question which, though ostensibly a sincere question for the purpose of gaining information, is asked for one or the other of two reasons. First, a child will ask a question designed to get the teacher started on a lecture during which most of the class may read some story book or magazine or look out of the window. The real nature of such a question is that of a protective measure, to keep the teacher from asking questions. The second is on the face of it absolutely sincere and even may be asked of the teacher privately, but nevertheless is a sign of resistance against instruction. The pupil is himself in this case unaware of his own resistance to taking knowledge in the place of getting wisdom. He really thinks he has a difficulty and sincerely feels that he desires to overcome it. But a little analysis will show that it contains a wish to put the burden of the work on the teacher instead of shouldering it himself.

This produces an unsatisfactory situation; for the teacher knows that to tell him what he consciously wants will not strengthen him but weaken him, and at the same time that to show him that his difficulty is one of his own making and unconscious wishing will put before him a conflict in which he will be quite unwilling to engage. Here, of course, the artless teacher, not reading the unconscious element of the pupil's situation, will give a long and painstaking explanation. The pupil will be gratified by seeing the teacher work so hard for him, but will not, of course, realize that the teacher is doing all the work and himself none, and, when a similar problem occurs again, the pupil will be little if any better able to solve it than he was at first. He will give it up then as a bad job, conclude that he has a special unfitness for that kind of problem and will hate it forever after, for he has, in his unconscious, come in close comparison with one who could do it a great deal better, and evidently took pleasure in demonstrating this power, while the pupil himself was inactive and unable to do a triumphant piece of work with it. His unconscious is tortured with a feeling of impotence and of envy of the teacher's superiority. If only a teacher's unconscious would let the teacher say sometimes that the teacher did not know! There might then be aroused a real emulation on the pupil's part to find out for himself.

The skilful teacher, on the other hand, will find out what are the real reasons for the pupil's being unable to fight out this battle for himself. His being unable to do it is of course not a true statement of fact. There are no students, or at most only a very few, who are really unable to do the work even of the wooden and senseless curricula now prevalent in schools. The inability is only fancied or phantasied, that is, wished for. The pupil really does not want to do that kind of work. He does not himself know that he does not wish it. The wish in most of these cases is an utterly unconscious wish. There may be even, and frequently is, a very strong compensatory conscious wish to do the work, or at any rate to get the reward for having done it, but interest in the work itself there is none.

When I say that the inability to do the work is only fancied, that is, wished for, I am implying a general identity between ideas and wishes.* There is in some pupils a strong masochistic tendency (see page 98) which leads them unconsciously to make themselves as miserable as possible over anything hard, being led thereto possibly by one or other masochistic parent, who takes pleasure similarly in bewailing the misery of human existence. The masochistic pupil will always look for and find difficulties and injustice where there is really none. He wants to be miserable, unconsciously of course, and finds ample opportunity in school.

---

* In general there is an absolute identity between a wish and an idea in one direction only. All ideas are wishes, but all wishes are not ideas. Perhaps it would be better to say that all ideas are the conscious elements of unconscious wishes, or that there is an unconscious wish as the cause of every idea which comes into one's head. Ideas of misfortune are no exception to this rule. That the wish is the father of the thought means just this: that no thought would occur to the mind that did not gain from the wish the motive power that drives it into consciousness. The very existence of an idea in one's mind is proof positive that there is a strong unconscious wish at the bottom of it. The idea would not have been vitalized, so to speak, without the dynamic force of the wish it contains.

Resistance in the Classroom

The phenomena of resistance to authority are seen in the actions of both teachers and children in school. The teachers forget the directions of the principal and the children forget the teachers' words, not only the commands, but also the words of instruction. This forgetting of the teachers' words on the part of the pupil is not because of any inherent inability to remember them, because retentiveness as a material quality is uniform in all persons, but because of the inherent nature of the relation between pupil and teacher. The teacher, due partly to the compulsory education law, where that is in operation, stands in a false relation to the pupil, i.e. a relation which arouses all the unconscious antagonism of the pupil. And that is why the problems of interest and attention and discipline are so puzzling. It is partly because the pupil does things all the time, prompted by the instinctive unconscious, and the teacher, with the usual rhetorical questions, asks *Why* have you done this? as if the teacher thought that the pupil could answer this question. It is perhaps a sincere thought on the part of some inexperienced and unreflecting teachers, but others must realize that the question is not really a legitimate one; not that there is no answer to it, but because the answer is impossible for all pupils and for most teachers.

The best attitude for the teacher to take is that which frankly implies that a certain number of acts have to be done, with the appearance of having to be done under authority at the command of a person who is supposed to be in authority.

How resistance against self-knowledge obscures the

judgment is illustrated by the following confession of a male high school teacher concerning the real causes of his giving more than the usual amount of attention to two girls, attractive, but not good students:

" On my way home from school after a séance with Miss X I reflected that I had possibly tried too openly to arouse her enthusiasm for her Latin, because her physical attractions had made such a reaction on my own unconscious. I had also taken the trouble to look up another very pretty girl to reprimand her for some irregularity in her classroom behaviour. I saw in these two facts the working of my unconscious desires and recalled that I had rationalized my acts at the time, giving as a reason for summoning Miss Y to my room not her pretty face with light hair and brown eyes, but the fact that she had given her place card to a boy to hand in and had gone up half a dozen points in so doing. I saw, as I walked home, the unconscious motives of both acts—the warming up about Latin with the one girl and the authoritative inquisition in the case of the other—and I realized as never before that I had been completely dominated in my choice of actions by virtually sexual motives. Furthermore, as I saw, after I had left the school building, that I would have given the wrong reason (had I been asked while I was doing those acts), instead of the true cause, so I realized that no person can possibly give the true cause for his acts, because it is hidden from him, and because, during the act, when he is most conscious of what he is doing, he is most unconscious of the real causes of what he is doing and so of the true significance of his acts. What, then, is the real meaning of any act? A real knowledge of one's unconscious can come only through a second person or from a second consideration of the act by the same person when he is in a different frame of mind, and is in a sense a different personality. The side lights on one's own character afforded by the remarks of another person, or even by the later study of one's own acts at a time removed from the heat of action, necessarily meet with a resistance directly in proportion to their truth, which must be painful and therefore repelled."

Resistance in the Market

Another illustration of resistance is that of having a smaller coin returned in change *under* and obscured by, a larger one, so that when one looks in one's hand one sees only the larger one, and, missing the smaller one necessary to make up the amount, one begins to suspect less change is being handed out than is due. This is a very prettily disguised bit of resistance on the part of the person making the change, because the change is all there and the salesman is just waiting for the purchaser to make an objection, which of course will be senseless. This will give the salesman a situation of superiority or at any rate that kind of superiority which comes from being wronged or unjustly accused by another. His remark to the purchaser will imply that the latter did not examine the change with sufficient care, certainly not with as much care as the change was arranged by the salesman. In that respect the salesman was truly the more careful and, in the detail of care, superior, and he gets much the same gratification out of the situation as he would out of any mild practical joke. All practical jokes hinge upon the sudden emergence of a situation in which the perpetrator is momentarily the superior, and " gets the laugh on " the other. But in the concealed coin " short change " trick above mentioned the resistance is very much covered but consists in the fact that it is a source of satisfaction to the salesman, who frequently in this episode is some small proprietor, even to appear for a short time, to give out less money than he should. Naturally he wishes to give back no change at all, but failing of this satisfaction, he unconsciously takes the next thing to it and gives for a moment the impression, both to himself and to the customer, that he is holding on to his money. The practical joke element of this incident is, of course, perfectly conscious. The salesman thinks that is all he wants, but fails to see the unconscious satisfaction taken by him out of the fact of the apparently retained money.

Transference as Identification

One of the ways in which identification works out is in the unconscious identification of a present personal relation with a past one. The individual behaves toward some person in his environment as he did toward his father or mother or their surrogate in his early youth. Roughly speaking this is expressed by saying that the school stands *in loco parentis* to the child. But the unconscious reaction to the parent in this relation has never been considered. That the school has taken up some of the functions of the parent is supplemented on the child's part by his unconsciously behaving toward the school, and more specifically toward the teacher, as he unconsciously behaved toward the parent. Thus an unfortunate home life, beginning even in the first year, will produce in the child either a rebellious, or a cowed, or a clingingly dependent attitude, for instance, which will be unconsciously and inevitably *transferred* to the teacher as the first person with whom he comes in close contact after father or mother. The transference is one of unconscious behaviour, and explains many of the child's reactions to teacher and, even at a later date, to some of his schoolmates. If the parent has been one of those who do everything for the child, thus interfering with his independence of action, it is quite likely that the same actions will be looked for from the teacher, who will find it most difficult to get any independent work done. If again the parent situation at home has contained an aggressive domineering father, it is quite possible either that the child, if a boy, will reproduce, through identification of himself with the father, the aggressive attitude toward the woman teacher, or the subdued and sullen attitude toward a strong man teacher. In any case the behaviour of the child in school is a replicá of that in the early home, or of the early influences.

Transference as a Means of Influence

This transference, however, which, it must be remembered, is absolutely unknown to the child, is the means by which the well-informed teacher can exercise the greatest good influence over the pupil. It will not be placed consciously before the pupil until the adolescent period is well under way, but, although it is something of which the younger pupil should never become aware, it should be consciously and systematically planned by the teacher, for it is his strongest card, not only to get efficiency in the petty details of school work, but also to exercise that much more benign influence which will give the pupil sureness and confidence in his behaviour toward reality in the years to come.

For the parent situation which tends to fix at an incredibly early age a pattern of behaviour in the child, the teacher is not, of course, in the least responsible. The parent situation, on the other hand, rather increases his opportunities for doing good, for, by means of the newer psychology, the teacher may acquire the power of consciously reducing this spiritual fracture and at the end of the course returning the child to the world much better equipped to meet its contingencies, though the pupil may never know it, than the school authorities or the state could ever expect.

A Wrangling Boy

As an illustration I might take a boy who lost his father at an early age and evidenced in the classroom a tendency to fly off the track at every opportunity. This was due not alone to the natural resistance to authority and to the accomplishment of work, for he had great ability, but was due to the habit he had unconsciously and blamelessly formed, of arguing with his mother. The teacher was at first dragged off the track and wrangled verbally with the boy, and then suddenly realized that he was himself reacting as the mother would have reacted in the same situation, and that here was a boy who had never had the opportunity of seeing how a rational man would behave toward a difficulty. The teacher then got control of the situation simply by refusing to follow the belligerent suggestions contained in the boy's unconscious attitude, and by showing him that there was no question of authority but merely one of the use of the boy's own very excellent abilities from which he could get a much greater satisfaction than from the discussion of essentially irrelevant topics with the teacher.

The Teacher's Transference

This illustration shows both the teacher's instinctive suggestibility to the attitudes of the children, which was fortunately overcome by the teacher's reflection about his own actions with the boy, and the fact that, without the deeper insight which the newer psychology gives into the unconscious behaviour of the pupil, the teacher might have been led far astray from the goal of education. It also shows that there is, in some teachers, at least, a transference of behaviour-pattern from the teacher's own home influence to the pupils in the classroom. Some teachers, in other words, are behaving toward their classes or to individual pupils in the modes to which they, the teachers, were initiated in their own infancy. Surely such teachers, at least, need the conscious attitude which the newer psychology can give, in place of that which they are unwittingly manifesting in their own reactions to the school environment.

Transference the Crux

The topic of transference is one of the most, if not the most, vitally important in the whole of the newer psychology. It is possible to give here only the merest sketch of its many applications not only in school but everywhere in human life. By a slight understanding of it teachers are immeasurably better able to interpret the otherwise frequently incomprehensible acts of children and adults, and themselves to react in a manner infinitely more serviceable to society than by blindly allowing their own transferences toward the children to control their teaching. But when it is realized how absolutely unconscious is this modelling of present behaviour on forms which were well fixed in infancy, it will be seen how impossible it is really to influence another soul unwittingly for its own good, without taking into consideration the unconscious elements of the general situation.

Any situation of human relationship contains, as I hope will be clearly seen by this time, elements of unconscious behaviour which practically control it and make it quite evident that all pupils and most teachers do not know what they are doing most of the time. Only by taking account of the unconscious element can they know all *they are actually doing.* Frink * has given a very clear explanation and Holt † one possibly still more apposite to the present topic, of the individual's unconsciousness of what he is really doing. Frink cites the instance of the retriever dog and how he is trained not to injure with his mouth the birds he retrieves, by means of giving him a bird stuck full of outward projecting pins. The dog mouths these very gently, and ever after retrieves *as if* he were carrying birds containing pins. The problem of analyzing out the transference element in behaviour of humans is to find, and in the case of adults

---

* *Morbid Fears and Compulsions,* page 508.
† *The Freudian Wish,* page 87.

get them to find out themselves, what are the " phantoms of past pins " to which they are reacting unawares.

" Phantoms of Past Pins "

If the teacher finds this out in the case of the pupil, he can act accordingly, without the pupil's knowing the significance of this action, and use the " pin phantoms " to improve his own work with the pupils. The realization of what are the " past pins," whose phantoms are such potent realities in his life, produces in the adult who is so fortunate as to discover them a truly rational reaction to the world of external reality which will remove most of his difficulties and enable him to use his entire force upon the world, unhampered by internal unconscious conflict. The dog was supposedly unaware that he was acting *as if* all the later birds were stuffed full of pins. We are all acting *as if* all the time, and the problem is to find out " as if " what. The solution of this problem is, I believe, possible for teachers. It is impossible for pupils, but unnecessary, if the teachers are themselves analytical enough to unravel their own past lives and unsnarl the children's for them, giving them only the net results in the shape of a new reaction pattern, which will help and not impede their progress.

Negative Transference

The concept of a negative transference is found to account for a marked hostility of the pupil to the teacher. In large schools with many classes of the same grade it is customary for a pupil who " can't get on " with one teacher, to be handed over to another. The process is sometimes repeated several times, with the final effect of branding the pupil as incorrigible, if he does not succeed in finding an agreeable teacher. This of course is a technical error and a loss of opportunity on the part of the first teacher who found the pupil impossible—a makeshift which allows a very interesting problem to go utterly unsolved. For the negative transference can, by the proper means, be readily changed into a positive transference in which the pupil's whole attitude toward life is likely to change for the better.

Transference and Resistance

As the concept of negative transference might by some persons be taken as one of the manifestations of resistance, it is necessary here to show the true relations between them. A negative transference, being an unconscious hostility to the person to whom the transference of the infantile pattern of behaviour takes place, remains nevertheless a transference. The expression of the emotional phase of it, however, is, by virtue of the ambivalent quality of emotion as such, invested in a negative form. This will seem contradictory to some persons, so I might illustrate from other sources. An artist is sometimes quite as pleased with a great deal of adverse criticism of his performance as with a small amount of favourable comment. Whether the comments are favourable or otherwise does not make so much difference as the fact that the performance causes a great deal of comment, which means that a great many people are much interested in it, or that their attention is compelled. Similarly of the child who is forced by an unconscious attraction to devote a great deal of attention to a teacher. The form that this attention takes is not as important as the fact of it. It may be wheedling, teasing, fawning, distant admiration or downright animosity. If the form it takes is displeasing to the teacher, it can be changed if the teacher knows how to do it. But in all these instances I am illustrating a transference to the teacher of an affection which once belonged to the parent exclusively.

Resistance is the only barrier to the outgoing of the soul to other persons and things and is based on inhibitions and fears. It is, like the other mechanisms, mostly unconscious, although it enters consciousness occasionally in the form of positive dislikes, the most patent form of resistance. Its latent forms may be inferred from many actions the characteristic trait of which is some defect. For instance, the absolutely innocent forgetting to do a school task, to comply with a request, even to think of doing a favour. In a certain sense no defective performance is absolutely innocent, on account of the resistance to doing a perfect performance, and we can hardly excuse the resistance. The very fact of its not occurring to the bridegroom, for instance, to take the wedding ring from the chiffonier and put it in his pocket, when he started for the church to marry the girl of his choice is an almost unmistakable indication of an unconscious resistance to marrying her. Not a single thing that we leave undone, except through sheer lack of time in an absolutely crowded life, is other than an indication of a resistance on our part against doing the very things we forget to do, or find insuperable difficulty or any distaste or disinclination whatever in doing.

This, then, shows the difference between transference and resistance. In some instances the pupil has no resistance against the teacher. He is only too anxious to plague. He has a transference for her, but it is a negative one. If he had the same degree of resistance against her that is indicated by the transference, he would forget her and her commands and requests, and his mind would be entirely engrossed in something else. She would be ignored. So any teacher can look around the classroom and make her inferences as to which pupils have positive or negative transferences for her and what others have merely a resistance against her. The latter will be the hardest to influence for their own good. In fact, some children are so brought up that they have a resistance against almost anything, particularly in school. The extreme degree of resistance renders the child ineducable.

Of course it may work out that a child has *a* resistance against doing a specific thing which happens to be the contrary of an act which would show a positive transference. For instance, a child does what he is told by his teacher, but gets it all wrong or, out of spite, does exactly the opposite of what he is told to do. Such an act should not be called a resistance. This negativism is the same as that seen in some insane patients who, when told to hold out the hand, will put it behind the back. They act immediately upon a suggestion, but negatively instead of affirmatively. Nevertheless they respond. In the schoolroom the lack of response shows the resistance, and it is the teacher's greatest problem how to remove it.

Medical and Educational Analysis

In the medical analysis used in the cure of nervous diseases the general resistance of the patient is effectually removed only by getting him to talk. Some practitioners believe indeed that the successful removal of the resistance perfects the cure, and that no cure is complete without the reduction of resistance to the minimum. In short, there is no topic which the patient should feel unwilling to discuss with the physician. A statement quite parallel to this could be made about the resistance of the child to the school environment. It will be found, in the school life of the child who shows a greater resistance than the average, that there is some thought which has occupied his mind to the exclusion of other thoughts and prevented the most helpful thoughts from being operative. In medical analysis the thoughts most obstructive are those which concern some thing which the patient has done and about which his conscience troubles him. It is safe to say the same thing about the resistant child in school, and also to say that the secret sin of the child can much more readily be confessed and much more easily condoned than that of the adult. But as it is the object of medical analysis to free the spirit manacled as it is with the inhibitions imposed upon it by a guilty conscience, so it is the object of educational analysis to release a spirit struggling against some obstruction which nine times out of ten is purely subjective or fancied. The resistance of the child against the details of the educational plan is based on his inhibitions, his fears. He fears that he may fail, that he may not get satisfaction and what not, and his fear, and thus his inhibition, should be removed so that he may get on a path where he may go ahead full speed without thought of error or harm.

The prospect of the teacher being able to free an imprisoned soul is a very inspiring one—almost as inspiring as the prospect of saving a lost one. But until today the way of doing this liberating work has not been thoroughly understood. In this of all times when most of the nations of the world are at war in the interests of political liberty, it is a proud thought for the teacher that he, too, although not privileged to taste of the consummate excitement of a life in the trenches, is nevertheless privileged to wage a war for freedom in every schoolroom in the land—the freedom of the human spirit from irrationality which is worse than ignorance. And just as the present war has developed new engines of destruction and a military organization embracing the entire world, so the most modern warfare of the spirit requires the help of the latest psychological discoveries, among which the one that stands out pre-eminent is that of the unconscious mental activity.

Summary

The attitude of the child toward work shows a perfectly natural resistance which is partly due to the authoritative manner of teachers. This produces on the part of the child an inability to express himself which in turn has developed a habit in the teacher of asking endless questions, whose insincerity prevents their being truly answered. The nature of a true question and a true answer is outlined. Teachers' questions are continued in spite of the fact that when the child fails to understand, his mind does not stop working, but proceeds to make and satisfy wishes in unremitting rhythm, of which the teacher is quite unaware, just as humanity in general is unaware of the unconscious wish-life of all individuals. Examples are given of the constant satisfaction of unconscious wishes by means of apparently senseless acts in school, both by mutilation of school property and by asking idle questions.

Other examples of resistance in the schoolroom are given, and one of resistance in the market. The transference of an attitude of the child from that maintained toward the parent to that maintained toward the teacher is described and examples are given, both of this transference and that of the teacher toward the pupil. Negative transference is distinguished from resistance. The relation between medical and academic analysis is noted.

CHAPTER VIII

EMOTION

AN emotion is the conscious or unconscious physical reaction to a stimulus which may be itself either conscious or unconscious. In one sense, then, we are having emotions all the time. But the further delimitation of emotions in order to separate them from sensations of the familiar "five" senses and the unfamiliar senses of weight, pressure, temperature, motion, etc., must include the specification that they are the mental reaction to a stimulus which is in the individual organism. The mental element, which is necessary to separate emotions from the purely physiological conditions which are continuous during the life of the body, has to be further qualified by saying that the emotions are not only a mental reaction to a stimulus which is in the body, but that the usually accepted emotions are those sensations which are most closely associated with the ego. In other words there are many sensations which come into consciousness, from the body, just as there are many sensations which are of too small a degree of intensity to enter consciousness, and these would be included in a definition which embraced all sensations of stimuli which were of internal origin.

I think that much would be gained by including all such stimuli, but then it would be hard to say anything about them or make any good inductions regarding them on account of indefiniteness. So, principally for the purpose of talking about what other people have meant when they speak of emotions, we have to cut out of the strict definition all those reactions to stimuli which are both of an unconscious origin and themselves of an unconscious nature, although we know that there must be such reactions to such stimuli taking place in the individual all the time.

Repressed Emotions

Furthermore we have learned in recent years that there are repressed or buried emotions that have an important effect upon the health of the individual, and that only academically can they not themselves be called emotions. There is no accepted name for them, and psychoanalysts have been forced to adopt a mode of description of them which declares that while there cannot be such a thing as an unconscious emotion, that is, an emotion consisting of the unconscious reaction to a stimulus which is either conscious or unconscious, and that therefore every emotion is by definition conscious, the actual original emotion of which the present emotion is but the substitute has not ceased to exist.

Thus, if a person has loved another and that emotion has turned to hate, the emotion called by the restrictive name love has ceased to exist, but this is quite analogous to saying that if a person has started to walk north and then changes his direction and goes south, then the direction of north has ceased to exist although the action of walking still continues. The emotion of hate may be the reverse direction of love, and yet the emotion may, as a unit which represents the original unit, persist.

Constant Quantity of Emotion

We have come to the conclusion that the unconscious craving for love, life and activity is constant in quantity, and that whenever it seems to disappear from the human consciousness it has not really gone out of existence but has, like a train entering a tunnel, merely disappeared from consciousness for a time. We therefore regard emotion as we regard the perennial vital urge, namely as continuous; and varying only in the degree in which it appears in consciousness. Just as we have desire all the time, we have emotion all the time, only some of it momentarily disappears from our consciousness to appear again at some later date.

What seems to make it necessary, in order to be consistent, that we should speak only of conscious emotion is the undoubted fact that we are never angry, for instance, at nothing.* When we *are* angry we are always angry at *something,* and that something changes from one thing to another. This condition we describe by saying that the ideational content of the emotion changes. This is not merely saying that when we are in good condition, physically, we think of now one thing and now another to be happy at. It means, on the contrary, that a flood of emotion, once released upon one idea or group of ideas, may meet with social opposition and become dissociated from those particular ideas. That does not mean, however, that the flood of emotion has been dammed entirely without outlet, for such a circumstance is as unthinkable as that any of the laws of physics should

---

* "In sooth I know not why I am so sad" may be spoken sincerely, but such a remark always denies the sadness or conceals its real cause.

all of a sudden be abrogated. But it means that the emotion once associated with one idea becomes associated
with another. A similar displacement is seen in the
sadism which (see page 89) has been repressed in its
natural original direction of pleasure at inflicting cruelty
to the direction of taking pleasure in having cruelty inflicted on self, or the other direction of preventing cruelty
from being inflicted by other persons upon still others,
where we have the anti-vivisectionists, and those devoting
a great deal of energy to the prevention of cruelty to
children and to animals.

From these considerations we infer that emotion is a
natural state of the organism, and that like respiration
and the circulation of the blood, it is variable only in its
incidence, by which I mean that just as the actual quantity
of the blood is the same, amounts of it supplied to the
brain, the muscles of the arms and legs, the stomach and
the intestines are different at different times according
to the exigencies of the organism, so the emotions are, or
I would better say, emotion is, a constant quantity, but
that it is, as it were, supplied to different ideas in different amounts at different times.

To carry the analogy a step further, if too much blood
is taken by the muscles at a time when there is food in
the stomach, digestion is delayed or made imperfect in
some way. In this we come very near home, because it
is well known that emotions, which exercise a deep influence upon the blood supply, will have the same effect
upon digestion. Some may say that I am arguing that
circulation is emotion. In a sense it is so, for both are
but forms of motion of the particles making up the body.
Circulation is sometimes " read off " into consciousness

and sometimes emotion is. Possibly it would be true to say that all physiological motion is read by consciousness now as circulation, now as sensation of the " five senses," and now as emotion. Here too the question of amount enters, for it is quite clear that a strong emotion so fills consciousness that there is room for little else and we do things of which we are not in the slightest degree aware.

So it adds to consistency of thought and logicalness of reasoning to regard all states of mind as conscious only in the degree in which they can, so to speak, be " read." That they are not read by the individual at any given time is no reason why we should have to regard them as non-existent. It might be clarifying to speak of a unitary " vitality " which comes into consciousness now as love, now as hate, now as the perception that the heart is beating violently, now as the perception that respiration is heavy, now as a pain in the intestines, now as a feeling of happiness and so on. This would be quite congruent with the principle which is taken as the fundamental hypothesis of psychoanalysis, namely, that the desire for life, love and activity is constant but subject to periodical obscuration, nevertheless continuing as long as the individual is alive.

But to return to the consideration of the emotions as such. The modern way of looking at them from the analytical point of view shows us things about them which at first sight seem quite contradictory. We hesitate to accept the psychoanalyst's dictum that militant suffragism is but the unconscious desire of the suffragette to be controlled by, and not to control, not men but a man, that the lynchings and the chivalry of the Southern States are not a desire so much to prevent outrage but to enjoy outrage. We might go to the extreme of saying that war is but an indulgence, in the part of every participator, of his propensity to inflict cruelty, but it would be unwise at the present time. Accustomed as we are to think in traditional modes of thought, we tend to object when we hear that self-sacrifice is only a disguised form of the desire to inflict cruelty upon others, transformed as it is into a desire to inflict cruelty on self, that love for women is a form of selfishness which differs only in degree from the love of anything else, and that emotions are but a kind of sensation differing in quality as does blue from the tone of a bell or from an actual pain of a cut finger.

If emotion is a form of human activity which is called emotions only when it is reported to consciousness through certain nerves that do not bring reports from outside of the body, and if the laws of this activity can be learned, then we shall certainly be in a position to act much more intelligently toward it in the classroom, in the home and in the world of business. William James put his theory of the emotions epigrammatically in saying that we do not cry because we are sorry, but we are sorry because we cry, but it certainly seems more sensible to say that we are sorry and we cry both for the same underlying reason, namely, that an unconscious mental activity is " read off " simultaneously by consciousness in two ways, as an emotion and as a flow of tears, just as an orange is read off as a colour and a fragrance, a touch, or a taste.

When the temperature of a metal is raised to a certain degree it gives off heat which is perceived by the sense of heat which is in the skin and mucous membrane. When it is raised to a sufficiently greater degree, it gives off light which is perceived by the eye. In a manner quite parallel to this we can say that when desire is raised to a certain degree it gives off emotion, and when raised to a sufficiently greater degree it gives off action.* Just as the metal when emitting light emits heat at the same time, so the soul when sufficiently stimulated gives off both action and emotion at the same time. It is not so very different if we say that just as heat is a mode of motion, so action and emotion are modes of motion, and the heat is a quality of both the material metal and the material animal body. On this analogy emotion becomes heat and action light, which puts the two in the accepted relation of value. Emotion in a person is metaphorically spoken of as heat, and as light is more valuable to society than heat, so is action more valuable than mere feeling. The social value of the action comes from its outward direction, and the comparatively smaller value of emotion comes from the fact of its inward direction. An emotion is a perception of something which is caused by an internal stimulus, and absorption of the mind in the emotions is an inward turning of the attention which if carried too far causes that form of introversion which leads to various kinds of mental morbidness.

Error of Extreme Idealism

An earlier philosophy chose to regard all experiences as they come through the avenues of sense as indistin-

---

* There we see temperamental differences in people because people melt or glow or boil or vaporize at different temperatures, the very reserved (=repressed) requiring the higher temperature.

guishable in the point from which they come. An extreme idealism would therefore look at every incoming sensation as merely incoming, and no matter how far it came, allowing no degrees of distance, making no distinction between impressions coming from the body itself and from the external world outside of the body. It was as if a person should sit and view the world through two panes of equally transparent glass. If there were nothing between those two panes of glass, such a manner of looking at the world would have no defect. But if there were a mass of animal tissue between the inner and the outer pane, which changed every ray of light coming from the world outside of the outer pane, it would make a great difference in one's reactions to the body between the panes and to the world of reality outside of the outer pane. To say that there was no difference in the appearance of the world viewed through the two panes is not the same thing as saying that no person can see the world without looking through them and what is between them. Of course he has to look through both and he has to infer that everybody else has to do the same thing. But a very practical result follows from the necessity of seeing through. If we delude ourselves into thinking that we can never see what is really there, outside of the two panes, we might just as well say that we cannot touch except by means of a jointed stick, which goes through the panes, the world which is outside of the outer one, and therefore there is no use in trying to act at all. Such a way of thinking virtually says: " Let us be content to stay in our glass case, for we shall never be able to go outside of it and wreak our strength on the real world which is out there."

The emotions are the things which nature has placed between the two panes of glass through which we have to see the world. Sometimes the emotions are cloudy and almost totally obscure the vision of things as they are, and sometimes they are as clear as any air and then we rightly think that we see things as nearly as they are as it is possible. But there has been little of value offered us by philosophy to enable us to clear the space of the cloudiness of the emotions or to maintain the bright golden hue which they sometimes impart to the world.

I have purposely chosen the figure of the two panes of glass to show its inadequacy. It is the view of an old and out-of-date philosophy. Put the entire human organism between the two panes, then take the two panes away, and what is the relation of the ego to the body and to the world? The ego is the body in every particle of its tissue and the world is external to it. There is no other way of looking at it. There is no difference between my self and my body, no difference between myself and my body and my mind. All are three ways of looking at the same thing.

The World as Part of the Body

But the opposite extreme of looking at the world as a part of the body is the way every infant begins his experience of life. He makes no distinction between the world outside of his body and that inside of his body, with the gradually beginning exception that he thinks all things which are painful are outside of and those that are pleasant are inside of his body. It is shown elsewhere in this volume how that innate tendency results in a habit of externalizing all unpleasant things throughout life and forms the mechanism of projection (page 118). But here I wish to emphasize the fact that the emotions are all sensations which do really emanate from within the body. Anger and fear are just as little a kind of stimulus coming from outside the body as are pain in the stomach or in a tooth, but both anger and fear are instinctively given an outward reference.

The paleontology of the emotions as we might call the analytic study of these mind activities, has shown that before there were any emotions there were only motions in the sense that a person in prehistoric times, if deprived of food by some other person, would not become angry at that person but would kill him, or get rid of him in some other way. Anger was first experienced by that prehistoric ancestor who was prevented from killing the other fellow and had to have some outlet for his activity. If he was held fast, say by some of his fellows, so that he should not kill the aggressor, who might have been a good warrior and consequently valuable to the tribe, he would have to bottle up his activities entirely or struggle with his captors until his desire for activity had waned. If in the long run he swallowed his wrath, his activity was spent on his own body. Probably he maimed himself, in lieu of the aggressor, actually tore his own hair and scratched his own cheeks, beat his breast or what not.

Anger a Self-Castigation

Nowadays the emotion of anger is nothing but a self-castigation which is practised by persons who feel aggrieved. It is practised on themselves because society, which is so infinitely stronger than it was, in those good old days when there were no Ten Commandments, has put a ban on doing those very retributive actions for which the instinct so loudly calls. So the modern individual, when attacked in one form or another, represses his rage, which is exactly equivalent to satisfying it on himself. Thus it is that anger is literally an " unfought fight." It is literally unfought in the external world only; it is literally fought in the body of the angered person. With weapons lying in his own body he slashes parts of his own body and does not see the extent of the damage. He only knows that he himself has been damaged, but what part of him and how he can have no knowledge. He attributes the damage, however, to the person who, he thinks, has injured him. He may have actually been wounded, and, had he been able to wound his enemy, he would not have given himself the internal gashes. There would have been two maimed men. Society gains, then, by restricting the damages to fifty per cent. of what they might have been and is thereby a great gainer in one way. But the man is the loser, because he has turned into a psychical wound what might have been merely a physical wound, and in modern times the psychical wound may be the worse. But society as a whole has not up to the present time been able to see that the mental is worse than the physical wound. Perhaps it is not. I shall not attempt to say.

I think, however, that I have illustrated what I wish to say about emotion. Not only is it a sensation of what goes on in the body, which might not have to be confined to the body if society had not put a ban on its being let out, but it is a sensation of a motion taking place in the body of which the individual has no other information than through analysis. He looks upon it as a strong feeling indefinitely located (or universally located all over his body), to which, however irrationally, he attributes an external origin. He thinks that the aggressor made him angry, or that the acts of the aggressor did so. But it is manifestly not the case. The aggressor did something to which there would have been a similar retributive action had not society restrained it.

Love an Unacted Caress

I have used anger as the illustration because the consistent carrying out of the retributive action would not so shock the sensibilities of the reader as if I had used love, which is so much more shocking than anger. If I should say that the emotion of love is but an unacted caress I should have been quite as logical. The aggressor of the preceding illustration becomes the lover in this, and so inconsistent is human nature that I should be considered too suggestive if I carried out the parallel any further.

We can be more detailed in illustrating the emotion of hope. According to the more modern view hope would be the unacted act of any description, the unseen sight, the unheard melody, all accompanied by a more or less strong desire. And as the unacted or unperformed act is really a performed act, but performed only within the organism and never let out into the external world of reality, it is quite plain not only that hope deferred maketh the heart sick but that it also makes the body sick as well, because it is but ungratified desire, or desire for outward experience gratified actually but gratified on the body of the desiderant.

Applying the same test to the emotion of sorrow we find it to be an unperformed wrong or an unacted tragedy. From this point of view one cannot sorrow long, rationally, because one realizes that an indulgence in sorrow for any length of time is but a rehearsing of the tragic, an acting of tragic scenes in our own ego. The element of desire is here quite as inevitable as everywhere else in human mental activity. If we sorrow for long, it is only because we have a desire to be sorrowful. It may be because we have a desire for the misfortune to overwhelm some other, the misfortune indeed for which we say we are sorry.

Naturally we should all wish to be joyful, and the emotion of joy, from the newer point of view, is but the enacting in the internal world of the body the acts which have been really acted or which we desire to act. It is evident how futile is joy of the second type, that enacted internally and projected into the future. If we give ourselves up to this kind of joy we become happy but introverted idle dreamers.

In all these illustrations we see the two elements of internally acted acts and of desire. But normal desire always is for externalization of activities. It is necessary for the organism perpetually to be taking things into itself from the outside and perpetually to be acting upon the outside world. Presumably the man of most continuous action most consistently externalizes all his acts and therefore has less emotion and less need for emotion than the inactive person. But this brings up the thought that there are many who are continuously active and who do not do the things which they most desire. In this case, of course, there is a conflict between what such a man wishes to do and what he does, and the conflict not only results in the detriment to what he is actually doing, because he is not doing it with all his heart,—that is, with all his desire; that is, with his whole body,—but it also results in the doing of what he wants to do at the same time but the doing of it in an internal manner. We all know how many clerks and other employees are doing one thing and dreaming about another, to the infinite harm of their work. We do not, and they do not, see the harm they are doing to themselves, but it is evident to all persons who think beneath the surface.

Education of Feelings

Education of the feelings, up to the present time neglected in favour of education of the intellect and to a less degree of the will, has been ignored partly from conscious and partly from unconscious causes. The conscious reason why the education of the feelings has been sidetracked is because it has appeared that the feelings do not play so important a part as the intellect in the practical work of the world. It is now seen that for a continually increasing number of persons (neurotics) the feelings play a part in their lives so important as to make them unable to perform their normal amount of work in the world. It is found that in these people the emotions of pleasure and displeasure, and the more dynamic passions of love and hate, are, by a twist that is primarily intellectual, transferred from ideas to which they really belong to other ideas which are not appropriate. It must be remembered that there is no feeling which is not attached to *some* idea, and while there are ideas which have no emotional tone, there is no emotional tone which does not belong to some idea. It is more or less like shadows and reflections. There is no shadow or reflection that is not the shadow of some object or the reflection of some surface. But there are certainly objects which, in the absence of light, throw no shadow, and surfaces which, because of their nature, can reflect no light.

The most recent psychological investigations have established the fact that a curious and very important transfer takes place between ideas and emotions. An emotion such as grief is felt first at the loss of a friend or relative or lover, and when it has become, or if it does become, too painful, it is repressed into the unconscious, that is, the idea or occurrence which originally caused the grief is repressed and the grief is attached to some other idea. One reasons somewhat as follows: This thought, of having lost this dear one, is so painful, if I could forget ever having known or loved him, it would enable me to forget the grief and be happy again. It is a fact that the memory of the loved person can be repressed into the unconscious, but if the organic basis of the emotion of grief is deeply enough founded in the system, the grief itself will immediately be linked up with some other occasion, and the individual suffering this change is forced to grieve over something else.

But the effects of grief which, like a scar, persist and are attached to some other idea, as if a man should have forgotten that his wound was received in a situation disgraceful to himself, and had pretended, and had come to believe, that the wound was received in battle while he was fighting bravely.

The effects of grief or anger are not so persistent or pervasive as those of love, and a person who has had a disappointment in love is suffering from a frustration of wishes that are fundamental in all humans. The love-desires, denied their gratification, continue nevertheless and attach themselves inevitably to another object if the first one is taken away, and this is the case whether or not these same love-desires have or have not been gratified before the final denial. In fact it may be said that while the wishes which form the core of the affection of love may be denied their gratification for days, months and even years, there is always a substitute gratification of them found in some form or other. If a man cannot marry his adored one and possess her fully, he will take some compensatory gratification from her caresses which convention does permit, and if the engagement is pro-longed beyond all practical limits, his desires of full pos-session of his fiancée will have to be gratified in some substitute form or he will lose his health of body or mind or both.

This substitution of one form of gratification of wishes is sometimes conscious. The man knows what he is doing when, inflamed by the beauties of his fiancée, he satisfies his gross sexuality on other women. But the case of women, or very much repressed men, is different. Wo-men are brought up almost universally to repress their sexuality in its franker forms. And so successful is this repression in what we call the most refined women, that when their fundamentally sexual wishes do come into consciousness, they appear not as sexual wishes but as wishes, desires, trends, bents of character, or keen interests so disguised as to be absolutely unrecognizable by the woman herself. One woman's desire for man's love and for maternity was so perfectly repressed that she developed a compulsion to take drugs, a feeling so strong as to compel her to take them constantly and indiscriminately, regardless of their nature. The poisons, of course, she took in medicinal doses. Her feelings so intense were transferred from where they really belong and where of course they are quite proper, to an idea (drugs) about which no such insatiable desires are proper. Her tendency to take drugs was absolutely unaccountable to herself and to everyone else until her mental life was inquired into analytically, when the real cause was found and the imperativeness of the feeling departed.

This woman was one of the numberless women who as children have had their sexual curiosity snubbed, and who have been carefully trained to repress all sexual feelings on the ground that they are base and disgraceful. Such women, in certain circumstances, can substitute other sensible and socially useful desires and interests in the place of those which their environment has suppressed, and can devote the energies which these desires express, to ends which bring a wholesome degree of satisfaction, to ends which, like that of reproduction, are creative, but are creative in other ways, such as art, literature or education.

But there is as yet no education which takes into account in any degree the greatest of all unconscious desires—the sexual. A half-hearted sort of instruction with averted gaze is given in some schools, and a few parents make futile attempts to instruct their children in sex, disqualified most of them by the shame they themselves feel about admitting the fact that they had and gratified sexual desires.

But how a boy or a girl should feel, much less how a man or woman should feel about the things concerning which the deepest and most pervasive feelings are right and proper, is very rarely considered until it is too late, and the sexual feelings which should be kept for sexual things, have gotten detached from those primal experiences and transferred to incidents which never in the world should have had attached to them feelings of sexual intensity.

In a sense, then, our civilization is based and the vast fabric of it is erected on a sense of shame, for repressed sexuality works itself out in excesses of every sort, in enormousness of cities, and commerce and all the great things which so astound the individual when he looks at them in large. It may thus be that our shame-civilization has resulted from a shunting off of power from reproduction of species to production of externals of life and that, had we had our sexuality less repressed, we should have been a simple people like the Chinese.

Unconscious Cause of Neglect

The unconscious reason for neglecting the education of the emotions, and for the neglect of the emotions in education, is that an emotion, being a purely subjective feeling, does not contribute any part to the activity of the individual that is directed toward the production of a change in external reality, but only contributes to a certain degree of intensity of outward actions. It both diminishes their effectualness at times, and at other times it increases the force of the outward impetus. But emotional action, or action largely motivated by emotion, is not in the long run as effective as that instigated by pure desire for activity, for it is, like emotion itself, most variable in its quantity, while the action motivated by the unconscious desire is normally—that is, if not blocked—continuous.

The deeper emotions are therefore to be regarded as an occasional accompaniment of activity, mental or physical, while the general affective tone of well-being or malaise, pleasure or displeasure, may be a constant undertone which seldom enters the focus of consciousness. A voluntary turning of attention to the emotions accompanying a thought or an action will either cause the emotion to vanish, or, if it seems to increase it, will do so merely by calling up other thoughts or evoking other actions associated with that emotion before. Therefore the individual who is not studying emotion from a purely psychological point of view is really trying in a purely introversional manner to use himself as a source of pleasure. The same is true of those who make efforts to maintain an unpleasant emotion. They are using themselves as sources of pleasure, only here they are deriving a masochistic pleasure out of the painful emotions. This is the condition of women who enjoy going to funerals, and crying about many other things. They identify themselves, as do all masochists, with the person who is getting pleasure out of the situation, the aggressor, and the enjoyment they take in the misery is that of the person inflicting the pain. The more wretched they feel, the more they enjoy it.

It is the same with children who exhibit too much emotion, as many do at home, about the learning of their lessons, and about their performances in the class. If a child is angered by being told he has made a mistake, or if he shows too much joyous excitement over having surpassed a competitor, he is too emotional. The actual expression of the emotion is not as significant as the existence of it, which the teacher may infer from the child's manner. The emotionality of such children is a very serious obstacle to their learning that for which they come to school. As has been mentioned (page 299), the emotion which upsets a child and makes him unable to understand his lesson is in reality a misplaced emotion. It essentially belongs to the more fundamental desires. It would be very advantageous if the teacher could find the opportunity to have a quiet talk with such a pupil, and find out indirectly, by means of inferences from his statements about apparently extraneous matters, what is the real unconscious thought at the bottom of the emotion.

The disproportion between the emotion as evinced by the child and that which would be appropriate to the situation is evidence enough that the emotion is misplaced. Its being misplaced proves that it belongs to an unconscious thought, and not to the conscious situation. The child himself has no knowledge of what the unconscious thought is, and he can never find out for himself. It is also quite unlikely that the teacher, if he found it out, could communicate it to the child directly. But the good result that will come from the quiet talk about the apparently extraneous matters is a new attitude on the part of each toward the other, partly at least due to their seeing more of each other. The child sees that the teacher is more than a mere critic, and the teacher that the child is more than a mere pupil. This fact alone will reduce the incident that has produced the emotion in the child to more nearly its proper proportion. If the child could see the incident in its truly normal proportion, he would not be so emotional over it. The emotion comes from placing a really trivial act in the position of a great tragedy, which implies a very narrow view of the act.

As to the extraneous matters mentioned above, I should here state that no matters that can be mentioned by the child are really so. He cannot talk of any topics which are not germane to the situation over which he became too emotional, unless the interval between the emotion and the quiet talk is so long that the thoughts connected with the emotion have time to become completely repressed. The quiet talk too should be mostly the child's and not the teacher's. "A quiet talk" from some teachers' point of view is really a long lecture by the teacher on the wrong done by the child, his duty toward school and parent, and the necessity that such a strong emotion or loss of temper should never occur again. This is not at all what I mean. On the contrary, the teacher should show such an interest in the child's life out of school as to lead the child to talk about himself, his likes or dislikes, his hopes or fears, his outside interests, anything in fact which will be apparently not connected with the emotion in question. I say apparently for the reason stated above that nothing that the child can say is irrelevant, being connected with the incident in question by the thoughts in the unconscious, all of which are pushed up to consciousness by the same unconscious craving which expressed itself in the over-emotionality.

The question of over-emotionality is important in many ways. The children who apparently have no emotions may be supposed to have the unconscious variety. The absolutely unconscious emotions probably have a deleterious effect, so that it would be better to get such children to express some emotion openly. This is one advantage of athletics in that it lets out emotions in some children who may not get the conscious emotion any other way.

Function of the Emotions

Have the emotions a function and if so, what? If they are but the entrance into consciousness of sensations having an internal origin, how do they differ from the ordinary, though not widely known, organic sensations, so-called? As listed by current psychology the organic sensations are those of motion, digestion, including hunger and thirst, circulation, respiration, sex, and position, also pain and pleasure. An emotion is any one of these mentally associated, not with anything internal, but always with something external or some thought having an external reference. In one sense an emotion is a pleasure or a pain, really having an internal cause but to which we attribute an external one. It is thought popularly to have an external cause on account of its being mentally associated with an external happening. But that does not make it really dependent on the external thing. If we always boil when we hear certain words we cannot truthfully say that the words are the cause of the boiling even though the two occur regularly together in our experience. For it is notorious that the regularity may be broken at any time and subsequently the relations reversed.

> *Vice is a monster of so frightful mien*
> *As to be hated, needs but to be seen*, etc.,

but the fact that this hate may change to love shows that there is no causal relation between the situation and the emotion. Many other things than vice may arouse at first one emotion and later on its opposite. But whether the one or the other, the emotion is all the time an internal sensation, for which we blame or thank some external situation or object. If I lose some money, my emotions are mentally associated with the money, though they emanate from my body. If I see some terrible thing, it is terrible to me only by virtue of the bodily reaction I unconsciously make to it. This reaction may be instinctive or educated, come from instinct or environment, from the unconscious as inherited disposition or as the result of environment, but it is still a reaction in my body and on it, and not a reaction having any immediate effect on external reality, though it may be said to have a remote effect on something outside of myself. For instance, the emotions aroused in me by being struck may have the result of making me strike back.

The expression " arousing emotions " indicates that the emotions are ordinarily asleep, that is, in the unconscious, where possibly they really belong, and are waked up and brought into consciousness for the purpose of preparing us to externalize our mental activity. If this preparation does what it seems to do, it increases the force of the desire, or focusses it upon certain objects, thus acting, in a sense, as a magnifying glass in changing the relative size or importance of some object in the field of vision. So the emotions enlarge the personal value of certain objects, and make now one and now another object or situation have such qualities for us that it becomes the object of our desire.

The unconscious craving always tends outward, but its natural extraversion is for the purpose of getting its own internal satisfactions. What definite things can satisfy it is settled only by the manner in which the body reacts to those things. Two main varieties in type of bodily reaction to external stimuli may be called dilation and contraction. Dilation is expanding to take in, read off by consciousness as pleasurable emotions, and contraction is shrinking, which has the same effect both of expelling what has been taken in and reducing the number of the individual's points of contact with the rest of the world. But the psyche can expand in one direction and contract in another, both at the same time. Thus come pleasurable emotions connected with one object and unpleasant ones with another. The fact that we may have opposite emotions in connection with one and the same thing at different times accords with the fact that the emotions are purely bodily sensations, and not some essential quality of the thing. Essential qualities of things are quite different in this respect from the emotional aura through which we perceive them. Stones are invariably hard and standing water is invariably yielding, and their qualities are constant for all normal persons. But the emotions aroused by Plymouth Rock or New York Harbour are different for different people, simply because the people are different. Thus it is that those who do not perceive that stones are hard and water is liquid are called idiots and those who do not thrill at the sight of historic stones or waters are not. The former perceptions cannot be taught; the emotions can be and always are.

Emotionality of the individual can be diverted from its original connection with the nutritive and reproductive craving (where it serves the purposes of self-preservation and race preservation respectively), and directed toward quite different activities. In fact emotion is the best, if not the only, means of disengaging the libido temporarily from its natural animal object and transferring it to an artificial and human object. Not until the magnifying glass of emotion is put before an object can it be truly said that the object has any significant existence for the individual. Emotion naturally connected by the nutritive and reproductive libido with certain objects is only through education, that is, artificially, associated with other objects. Then for the first time do those objects come into being for the particular individual.

Thus it is evident that the only way in which to cause things to exist for the developing mind of the young person is to insure their being connected with an emotion of the expansive type. If they are by some inadvertence or ineptness on the part of the teacher allowed to become associated with the opposite type of emotion, their possible existence is annihilated so far as the particular individual is concerned. Being connected with the expansive (pleasurable) type of emotion is analogous to a situation where the given object would cause in the individual a bodily reaction of the dilation or acceptance variety, although it cannot be said in any true sense that the object is the *cause* of the emotion. For it is a fact that there are few if any instinctive emotions not connected with the nutritive or reproductive libido. Young children have no sense of disgust, for instance, for many things which adults have, and those instincts which apparently connect certain sensations with displeasure, such as the sensations from wine and tobacco, are subject, through education, to a complete reversal. Wine, which was unpleasant, becomes pleasant, and for a great many persons milk, which was the most desired object, becomes one of the least desired.

This dirigibility of the emotions, this fact of our being able to cause the reactions originally responding to one kind of object or situation to respond to another, is what makes education possible, because it makes the possibility that the second kind of object may have an existence or meaning for the individual, a meaning which otherwise, that is, without this transfer, would not exist. The transfer, however, is one of object and not one of response to an object. The response is the same, but the object is changed. Here the true nature of sublimation emerges into view. The two phases of the libido, if they adhered constantly to their original objects, the objects with which sex and hunger are satisfied, would be the same in humans as they are in animals. But humans have the privilege of devoting these two phases of the race-preservative and self-preservative libido to other objects than those instinctively suggested by nature, and therefore the privilege of having more objects in the external world have a meaning for them. This meaning or significance is a widening of intellectual vision through the magnifying lens of emotion, and is in effect really an amplification or magnification of the individual through purely intellectual means.

An Absorbing Interest in School Work

A child may be and must be taught to take the same degree of pleasure in absorbing knowledge of the objects of the external world and the relations between them that he takes in eating. The nutritive libido must and can be engaged upon a sum in addition with the same abandon with which it is engaged upon the sucking of a lollipop. Where this unity of effort, this focussing of the entire libido upon the sum in addition is not secured, it is safe to say the emotional magnifying glass has not been used by the teacher for the pupil or has been unskilfully used. Mostly the teacher holds the glass up before his own eyes and tells the children how large the object appears to *him,* not taking the trouble or not being mentally capable of finding out whether the glass is in front of the child's eyes or not.

It will require the teacher to have a knowledge of the unconscious mental activities of the children, for him to know whether the children have any appreciation of the meaning of what both teacher *and* children are saying. Many times the child will make what sounds like an intelligent remark and is accepted as such by the teacher. The next remark of the child will, if it is made, show that he completely misunderstands. Generally, however, it is never made, and the teacher loses the chance of making the comparison between the two remarks, a comparison which alone will reveal the unconscious thought connecting the two remarks. This is a crucial point. The child should desire to make more than one remark about the subject, just as he naturally sucks more than once on the lollipop.

Continuance of Activity

There is the same unconscious motive *possible* for the continuation of expression in words as there is for the continuance of the sucking, but the emotion of pleasure has not only not been connected by the teacher with the verbal expression, but in most cases it has been disconnected. While the child should desire to continue efforts in the intellectual sphere just as he naturally pursues activities in the absorbing of candy, he is prevented solely by the conditions of his educational environment, by the practically prohibitive attitude of the educational authorities, due to their ignorance of the mechanisms of the unconscious mental activity. The curriculum is fixed and the syllabus is prescribed and the work of the educational leaders is *done* and cannot be changed. The effect of the present academic environment *must* be inhibitive because it has produced the present results, comparatively good though they may be, for it is inconceivable that truly appropriate emotional conditions would not allow the pupil to devote as much libido to school work while he is in school as he does to extra-mural work and play *while he is out of school.*

Engagement of Libido

The fact is that the pupil's libido is not thus engaged. In other parts of this book I have tried to show both why it is not so engaged and upon what it is engaged, namely upon unconscious thoughts and actions, because of the virtual prohibition of the connection between the libido and conscious activities. In this section I have tried to show the means, that is the emotions, which may be used for the purpose of connecting the libido with the school activities. The school activities, in short, are not and they cannot be natural to the child. In lieu of naturalness, their artificiality, which is essential because the very aim of education is in a sense to improve upon nature, is one which will not be completely successful unless all the factors entering into the situation are accounted for. Up to date the greatest of all these factors, the unconscious, has almost universally, through unavoidable ignorance, been left out of account.

Education of Emotions

The question then arises concerning the education of the emotions of the child in the school. It is an undoubted fact that many if not most teachers, by their wholesome attitude toward the work which is to be accomplished in the school, produce the best atmosphere for the natural development of the normal emotions. There is, in the presence of such a teacher, neither too much emotionality nor too little. The work is personal enough, but not too personal. The appeal to the individual child is sufficiently intimate, but not too close. But the conscious and systematic treatment of the problems coming up in both the home and the school has not been accomplished according to the most modern information about the facts of emotion. Indeed it is safe to say that the problem of the emotions of the child has not appeared in its present-day light in school education at all. To go at the thing directly would be most artificial. For of all mental states an emotional one is the one which *par excellence* changes, and changes essentially, if attention is bestowed on it.

The education of the emotions, so useless to attempt consciously in the sense of arousing the consciousness of the pupil to them, must be done consciously by the teacher only. He must be instructed in the indirect means of getting the best emotional atmosphere in the pupils and without their knowing that they are being led in any direction in this field. This applies to pupils under the age of adolescence. To those who are passing through the adolescent period, some knowledge of the fundamental sources of emotion should be imparted. This is the only place where conscious efforts on the part of the teacher should be made to produce a conscious effect on the pupil. How this should be done is a question which cannot be answered here for lack of space. I have briefly indicated elsewhere (page 185) how some of the questions deeply affecting the emotional life of the very young child should be answered by the parent. But the emotional effect on the child at the time of the occurrence of these questions is almost nothing. That on the parent may be very great, according to his or her bringing up, but it has been found that questions of sex, when left unanswered, or answered in the traditional mendacious way, keep coming up again and again in the child's mind even to a date much later than is generally supposed, while the sincere and truthful answers given by the mother to the very young child about the origin of his life have the effect of once and for all dismissing any doubts and queries from his mind, and he is enabled to go ahead with the business of his child's life without the undue emotionality which is caused by unsatisfied curiosity about sexual matters.

The Aim in Education of Emotion

The principal aim in the education of the emotions is to get them placed on the right ideas. A child that weeps about a lesson, whether during its preparation or after its criticism by the teacher, is a common example of misplaced emotions. The deep emotions of the child should be aroused only about the most vital things. And as the most vital things do not normally concern the child, and only unconsciously concern him at the age of adolescence, the emotional child is one who has not had the proper bringing up at home. A child should not, either, take too much pleasure out of the successful achievement of his school tasks. If he does, it implies that things which so unduly excite him do so because he has been somehow, either at home or in the street, unduly excited sexually. For this the teacher is of course not responsible, but it is the teacher's duty to recognize the fact, and act accordingly, which will mean that he should, in cases like this, take particular care to avoid excitement of any kind in too great intensity, and endeavour to see that the child's life in school shall proceed as equably as possible.

Self-Abuse

In short, only the milder emotions should be aroused in school life. In a sense, therefore, the education of the emotions is not a school affair, except in the matter of the more superficial ones. But after the period of adolescence has set in, the question is one which cannot be excluded. In the earlier years of school education, the training of the emotions should therefore be negative. The traces of major emotions which crop up in school should be noted and the child exhibiting them given special attention for the purpose of reducing them, as a surgeon might reduce a fracture. For an outburst of emotionality on the part of a pupil is much like a fracture. A bad one is the opportunity for the teacher to go at the case consciously with that pupil alone, in order to find out the true cause, and by learning of it removing it, particularly if it is a case of unsatisfied or wrongly satisfied sexual curiosity, or of masturbation. The latter is as natural and inevitable in most children as is the tendency on their parts to think that they themselves are the only ones in the world who have discovered this source of gratification, and to think that because of that isolation they are outcasts, weaklings and doomed to an early death. As it is a known fact that self-abuse is common in all children of both sexes and at different times from the earliest infancy, and that a great amount of later neurosis is due to the false ideas which the children get of its injuriousness, it is particularly important for teachers as well as parents to know that the injury received from the indulgence is frequently if not always less than that received from the child's brooding over the secret sin, and his generally erroneous inferences about its effects. Such children, if not set straight about this matter, either by parents, who very seldom convey the correct information, or by teachers, are the ones in whom the major emotions have been initiated too early and at the same time not reduced, as the correct information about this matter generally has the effect of doing.

Mental Self-Abuse

While on this topic of self-abuse and the heightened emotionality which it produces in the life of the child, which some might compare to the lighting of a fire in a place not yet prepared for a fire of such magnitude, it will be appropriate to call attention of teachers and parents to the symbolic self-abuse which is existent in all over-intense emotionality in children (or adults too, for that matter). A great amount of pleasure which children take out of doing some habitual thing, such even as eating of candy, and sucking of lollipops, chewing pencils, putting hair in mouth, scratching head, stroking hands and neck, anything in fact which becomes an accentuated mannerism, is likely to be carried on by the pupil for the gratification of an unconscious desire which is essentially masturbatory in its nature. Such children are getting pleasure out of themselves, and not, as they should, out of external realities. It is very easy, comparatively, to change the habits of children. If allowed to go on till after adolescence these habits are very hard to break up, and they invariably indicate a certain degree of introversion. Teacher or parent must see to it that the child is absorbed not in himself, for he will get satisfaction of unconscious desires somehow, but in the world of external reality. This is the problem of the teacher and parent with many nervous children. Some of them are showing a tendency to become introverted, the bashful, the diffident, the retiring, the unusually quiet children, the omnivorous readers. They all use their own bodies or minds to a certain degree, in lieu of the world of external reality. It is inevitable that this should occur in all persons to a moderate degree; it is only the excessive or exclusive use of self as the world which demands corrective measures at once.

The use of one's own mind as a world on which to expend one's mental energy is, to be sure, far the best form of self-abuse, but is nevertheless undoubtedly a variety of mental masturbation. In the ordinary parlance daydreaming is the term applied to this mental activity. In the analytical psychology it is called " undirected " thinking or " phantasying." Its essential characteristic is the securing of the gratification of unconscious wishes by the easiest means, namely on the self. It is the satisfaction of the unconscious desire in the instinctive way. It is furthered by the reading of light fiction and attendance upon light drama. As the word " day-dreaming " indicates, it is, like the night dream, the ideal fulfilment of the wishes of the unconscious, voluntarily allowing whatever thoughts occur to have free play in the mind. Naturally the tendency in some persons is toward the frankly erotic, and in others toward the slightly disguisedly erotic.

Every child in every schoolroom who pauses too long from the assigned work, and sits rapt in inward attention, is excluding the external world. which has become irksome, and is retreating into self for the sole purpose of gaining a satisfaction which it does not know how to secure in the world of external reality. This is the teacher's chief concrete problem, then: to show how satisfaction can be gained from the world of work, from the definite tasks allotted in the schoolroom, and from the interplay of personality between pupil and classmate and teacher. The pupil's gaze is to be directed outward instead of inward, and forward instead of backward.

Forward instead of backward here has a double sense, for the pupil, in introverting, as this selfward-directed activity is called, is regressing mentally to the age in which the satisfactions are normally taken out of self and not out of the external world, namely, the age of infancy. This is not to say that regression is a defect at all times, for the most active minds have their normal periods of regression; for instance, the noted men who occasionally relax in reading dime novels or other cheap literature. The universal normal regression is of course sleep, where the individual goes back into pre-natal oblivion and opens the door for any kind of phantasy.

Education of the Will

From the point of view of the newer psychology there is little to be said about the will. I have spoken about the battle of wills which takes place occasionally in the schoolroom. The same frequently takes place in the home between the parent and the child. The fact of two human wills opposing each other has an aspect of a degree of economic folly that is almost pathetic to witness. When we multiply this war of individual wills into a war of nations like the present, we see very clearly the unnecessary destruction which it causes. But in the single struggle between two wills, when it is about the will alone and not about something toward which the will is directed, when, in short, one will is directed against the other will, there is a displacement of libido which is extremely unfortunate for humanity as a whole. For of the two directions of the individual will—namely, the direction of it upon another will or upon a *thing* in external reality— there is no question whatever as to the greater advantage of directing the will toward things over directing it against persons.

With respect to the education of the will, the newer psychology teaches that the will does not have to be educated or trained any more than a stream of water or a pressure of steam, implying that what is called weakness of will is really a blocking or damming of the libido by the inhibitions caused by the complexes, and that, instead of training the will, as a weak muscle is strengthened by exercise, the libido has to be liberated and it will exert itself to its maximum, like any other unimpeded natural force but on socially approved objects.

Those children in school who appear to have weak wills, if they be not of a congenitally weak physical constitution, have naturally just as strong a will as the most assertive and obstinate child, but their will, or more accurately, their libido, has been blocked by some fear or other inhibition, which is caused either by a guilty conscience about sexual matters, generally utterly unwarranted guilty feelings, or by one of the phases of the family complex. So it would be particularly happy if, through the teacher's knowledge of the unconscious wishes, that are working in such a tangled way in the hinterland of the pupil's mind, the child's fears could be removed and he could be given the confidence to go ahead full speed. As a very concrete instance of a parental influence operating against school work I might mention an almost pathetic child in the first primary grade who could not handle a pencil. His father, in order to get fun for himself out of Johnny's first day in school, had told the boy that he had better look out for the pencil because it would bite him, and hence the poor child's efforts to write were impeded by his thought that he had to handle it most gingerly. The inability of most children to do well in any given study is determined entirely by the unconscious preconceptions which they have formed about the difficulty or impossibility of their being able to reach a standard set for them, and not because of any " weakness of will " or stupidity in understanding the subject. It will be different in different cases. What the teacher has before him is generally not a weak will but an obstructed will, and it takes an analytical examination of the individual pupil to get at the bottom of the trouble and remove the obstruction. This cannot be attained without the previous establishment of a rapport between himself and the pupil, analogous to that existing between the physician and the patient in the medical psychoanalysis. It implies a transference of the right kind on the part of the pupil toward the teacher, which cannot be produced unless the teacher is able to read below the superficial manifestations of the pupil's conscious thoughts and acts.

Here, then, is the teacher's, as well as the parents', real opportunity. The thoughtful parent, who has the leisure and the interest, will occasionally study the unconscious of the child, when his or her attention has been called to the existence of such a thing. It is the *duty* of the teacher, and the sole art of teaching, to produce an effect upon the pupil without the pupil's knowing how it was done. To this end the teacher will have to gain the confidence of the pupil to the extent of the pupil's telling the teacher a great many of his thoughts on subjects apparently most remote from the subject of study in which the pupil appears to be weak in understanding or in will. In these talks the child will, in most cases, reveal to the discerning teacher acquainted with the mechanisms of the unconscious, the real cause of the apparent weakness of will, or of the seeming lack of intelligence. The teacher will discover the true reason why the unconscious of the child is unwilling to see or understand, or thinks he is unable to do so, and will be able in many cases to throw a bright light into regions which were for the pupil dark before.

Summary

Emotion is described as the perception of a stimulus that originates within the body, but which has a closer relation than other sensations so originating with the apparent desires of the individual. While it originates within the organism it is referred outward, as ordinary feelings of discomfort are not, and is associated with some more or less definite idea. The existence of repressed emotions suggests that emotion is a constant factor of all mental activities, which appears in consciousness with greater or less intensity according to circumstances. Emotion is likened to a coloured medium through which the external realities are perceived. Extreme idealism regards even the external world as a part of the ego. Anger is shown to be a form of self-castigation, love an unacted caress, and analogous statements are made about other emotions. The education of the feelings is based on the fact that the idea originally associated with the emotion may be changed for another idea. The function of the emotions in school is to further continuity of activity, the education of the emotions in school should be indirect and the unduly deep ones reduced wherever possible. The connection between emotion and the sexual life of the child brings up the question of physical self-abuse, the dangers of which are explained and the question of mental self-abuse, which is too common among children in forms least suspected by teacher and parent. The education of the will is merely the removing of obstacles existing in the unconscious.

CHAPTER IX

CONCLUSION. MEDICAL ORIGIN

A SPECIAL significance attaches to the fact that the strictly scientific method of studying the unconscious has come from medical research. The first authoritative result was reached by a neurologist in searching for the causes of a nervous disease. Having found it in the unconscious wishes, the unperceived tensions existing in the mind of his patient, he was quick to see the application of his discovery to all phases of mental life, normal as well as abnormal. For the only difference between normal and abnormal is the fact that the so-called abnormal person finds a difficulty in living in society. Society shows him up for abnormal only by setting standards of adaptation to which he is for some reason unable to measure up.

Education is the conscious effort on the part of society to lift as many individuals as possible up to the standard which it has set. Therefore any knowledge of the reasons why some do not naturally rise to or above such standards is welcome, no matter what the source. And any knowledge of the means for such an uplifting of the individuals who are below the average is doubly welcome.

In this connection it may be of interest to give a slight

idea of the methods pursued by the medical psychologists in the cure of certain nervous diseases.

Medical Psychoanalysis

Those physicians who confine their practice exclusively to cases where psychoanalysis is available for the cure of diseases of a nervous character have summed up their work by saying that at bottom it is really a process of educating the adult to adapt himself to the requirements of his environment, an adaptation which has been unsuccessful. The failure to adapt has been the cause of the disease which the patient has sought the physician for the purpose of curing. The methods of these physicians, which in the rarest cases include the prescription of drugs, vary within certain limits, as it must according to the mental development of the physician himself. Ostensibly the method is to evoke, by patient listening, the apparently trivial thoughts which the patient may have during the hours which he spends with the physician, so that the general trends of the unconscious craving may be diagnosed, and the appropriate counsel given. Some physicians give advice about concrete matters concerning the patient at every sitting, thinking that otherwise the séance may have no point for the patient, while others will receive and listen to the patient for weeks at a time without offering a single suggestion, on the theory that knowledge which is applied by one person to the surface of another is merely superficial and has no dynamic value, which is gained solely by the patient's making his own inferences. In one sense, as has been already said, it is a physical impossibility to tell anybody anything, particularly about himself.

But the general aim is to educate in the sense of bringing out all the capabilities of the patient in any and every line, so that after mature reflection, and the necessary spiritual growth, which time alone can effect, he will be in a position to make the correct reactions to the stimuli which constitute his environment.

The gist of the lesson which the patient learns is what he is actually doing in his everyday life, for on a knowledge of what he *is* doing must be based the determination to do what he ought to do. It is always found that the patient is unwittingly doing something that is not approved either by himself or society. What he should do is what society, in the broadest sense of that term, requires of him. He may think that he is doing exactly what he is required to do, but in this case he is deceiving himself and the self-deception has to be revealed to the patient by the physician. This implies that conscience is the determining factor in the origin of many diseases of nervous character, the conflict between what the patient thinks he is doing and what he thinks he ought to do being the crux of the whole situation. When the patient is deceiving himself both about what he ought to do and about what he is doing, it is evident that he is far from adapting himself to his environment in the most constructively social way.

A concrete illustration * of the way in which the patient suffers from a conflict between himself and society is that of the woman who became a nervous wreck from thinking that the people of the suburban town where she

* Frink, *Morbid Fears and Compulsions,* page 157.

lived after the death of her husband were unfriendly and critical to her because they thought she was a designing widow, and was making eyes at every available man. She had to be taught that in the first place she was actually at heart what is called a designing widow, as she really wished to get married again; and then, on top of that, she had to be taught that it was no crime to get married again, anyway. This rather amusing way of putting what was a source of intense conflict to the unhappy woman is a good instance of how the aim of psychoanalysis is to make us see ourselves as others see us with the implication that when we do we shall react as others do in the same circumstances, and that if we do so act we shall be free from the conflict which is the cause of our misery. And our misery, however purely mental it may have been in the beginning, sooner or later, if our warped view of ourselves and our relations with others is not corrected, will become a physical ill, which will respond but weakly to physical means of remedy, as it is really of mental origin and can be eradicated only from the mental side.

So that the aim of psychoanalysis, whether it be the corrective work of the physician or the educator, is the same. It is to unite the individual with his kind. It may be said that there are many people in the world who are perfectly united with their kind but who are not educated. But it will have to be admitted that such people are really, in a broad sense, better educated than the college man with the highest degree, who cannot in spite of it be happy himself or live happily with his neighbours. He may be educated, but he has only a specialized form of training and has not the education which is of most worth.

I hope that if I can call the attention of my fellow-teachers to the very much more social way of looking at their calling which the psychoanalytic view presents, I shall be able to make the work of the teacher more efficient, his relations with parents and children more profitable and his position in the present social organism more valued than it is.

FINIS

INDEX

Printed and bound by CPI Group (UK) Ltd, Croydon, CR0 4YY

01/11/2024

01782630-0007